Good Practice in Psychodrama

This book is dedicated:

To Jeanne, my wife, a friendly and admirably perceptive reader of my text in preparation.

To my family.

To the memory of Dr Dean Elefthery, consultant psychiatrist/psychotherapist and psychodramatist.

To Doreen, his wife who survives him, actor and psychodrama trainer/practitioner and director of the International Foundation for Human Relations. Dean and Doreen were my primary trainers.

To all the members of my training group who shared with me.

To all the trainees I have worked with as their training director.

To all the clients, colleagues and patients of my psychodrama therapy groups, many who appear in this book in other guises.

THANK YOU.

Good Practice in Psychodrama
an Analytic Perspective

DON FEASEY

Analytic Psychotherapist (UKCP Reg), Manchester

W
WHURR PUBLISHERS
LONDON AND PHILADELPHIA

© 2001 Whurr Publishers
First published 2001 by
Whurr Publishers Ltd
19b Compton Terrace, London N1 2UN, England and
325 Chestnut Street, Philadelphia PA 19106, USA

All rights reserved. No part of this publication may be
reproduced, stored in a retrieval system, or transmitted in
any form or by any means, electronic, mechanical,
photocopying, recording or otherwise, without the prior
permission of Whurr Publishers Limited.

This publication is sold subject to the conditions that it
shall not, by way of trade or otherwise, be lent, resold,
hired out, or otherwise circulated without the publisher's
prior consent in any form of binding or cover other than
that in which it is published and without a similar
condition including this condition being imposed upon
any subsequent purchaser.

British Library Cataloguing in Publication Data
A catalogue record for this book is available from the
British Library.

ISBN: 1 86156 213 6

Printed and bound in the UK by Athenaeum Press Ltd,
Gateshead, Tyne & Wear

Contents

Foreword vii
Preface ix
Introduction xiii

Chapter 1 1

Historical overview

Chapter 2 11

Psychodrama is group psychotherapy

Chapter 3 29

Learning in the psychodrama therapy group

Chapter 4 43

What can and cannot be achieved

Chapter 5 55

A diagrammatic description of psychodrama

Chapter 6 61

From thought and feeling into action

Chapter 7 77

The art of psychodrama

| **Chapter 8** | **91** |

Interlude

| **Chapter 9** | **101** |

The protagonist

| **Chapter 10** | **115** |

Members working together

| **Chapter 11** | **125** |

The unities of time, place and person

| **Chapter 12** | **135** |

The psychoanalytic presence

| **Chapter 13** | **147** |

Ethical issues

| **Chapter 14** | **155** |

What next?

Conclusion	**159**
Bibliography	**161**
Index	**165**

Foreword

Jean Vanier, in *Becoming Human*, states

> The heart, the metaphorical heart, the basis of all relationships, is what is deepest in each one of us. It is my heart that binds itself to another heart; it leads us out of restricted belonging, which creates exclusion, to meet and love others just as they are.

The concept of encounter is in the centre of the group process. J.L. Moreno defined encounter as:

> A meeting of two
> Eye to eye
> Face to face
> And when you are near
> I will tear out your eyes
> And place them instead of mine
> And you will tear out my eyes
> And place them instead of yours
> Then I will look at you
> With your eyes
> And you will look at me
> With mine
> (Moreno, 1934)

This is role reversal: a way to really meet oneself and the other person, a way to touch the heart within the role. It offers an opportunity to become and remain alive, in a society where we relate to each other increasingly not as human beings but as object to object, and often without respect for the dignity and freedom of the other. We are in danger of becoming friendly users in a 'user friendly' society. Role reversal can help keep the 'I–thou' relationship alive.

Don Feasey's aim 'to draw psychodrama closer towards the creative development of psychoanalytically influenced psychotherapy and counselling, as it is used in [England] today' could be a great asset to many people in the helping professions. Psychodrama is used effectively as an extension of the group process in many other countries.

Moreno, a psychiatrist, intended psychodrama to be part of a triad with group psychotherapy and sociometry. In the United States, in the 1960s, psychodrama moved away from group work and sociometry, when many people were carried away by the action of the drama. However, the psychodrama director is not a theatre director, and the audience is not the audience of the Renaissance theatre. Therefore, psychodrama was often misused by people who confused the role of director with theatre director rather than a therapist facilitating a process, with as much emphasis placed on the working through as on the catharsis.

Moreno may have had a flamboyant personality but his heart was always with his patient's heart and his knowledge as a clinician was obvious. He emphasized that psychodrama was as much a method of restraint as of expression, should only be in the hands of qualified people, and should always be used with respect for the freedom and dignity of every individual member of the group.

Dean Elefthery always cautioned therapists to ask themselves 'whose need is it?' when moving from the group discussion phase to the overt action phase in a therapy session. A knowledge of sociometry allows one to read the depth dimension of the group and helps to protect one from being unconsciously manipulated by the group dynamics and/or one's own unconscious, to move from the role of isolate (facilitator) to 'star' (theatre director).

The gift that Freud, Jung and Moreno have given to us includes their daring action of the mind, and their courage to step outside the norm, and to find, within their own creativity, a way to integrate their fellow man into a more meaningful way of life.

Don Feasey, with his sound knowledge of theatre and many years of experience as a therapist, offers a challenge to his readers to step outside their norm. He offers a new approach, a way back to the heart 'out of restricted belonging which creates exclusion'.

Doreen Madden Elefthery

Preface

The presence of psychodrama as a therapy and a theory has gradually impinged on the mental health scene in Britain. Its presence has come late and tentatively, largely because it has been seen in the past as a rather florid form of American psychotherapy associated with encounter groups and west-coast exhibitionist therapies. Actually, psychodrama came from Europe at about the same time as Freudian psychoanalysis and, in some respects, rivalled it in those early days. Like psychoanalysis, it was taken up with enthusiasm in America, and Moreno, its inventor, went to live and to practise in America where he was celebrated. From his emigration to America has come, in its maturation, the influential and respected American Society for Group Psychotherapy and Psychodrama.

My aim in this book is to draw psychodrama closer towards the creative development of psychoanalytically influenced psychotherapy and counselling as it exists in Britain today. The last 10 years have seen a great growth in psychotherapy and counselling and the influence of Rogers and Freud is paramount. During this time psychodrama has arrived and a number of training centres have been set up. The most influential centre has been Hoewell in North Devon where Marcia Karp, a graduate of the main American centre and a Fellow of the American Society of Group Psychotherapy and Psychodrama, came to work in the 1980s. The arrival of Moreno inspired psychodrama in this country, just as psychoanalytical influence began to re-emerge with increasing force and influence, producing a certain tension between the different schools of thought. Moreno, although inclined to messianic mysticism, was clearly of the humanistic therapy culture. American 'ego' psychology had played its part, too, in influencing the development of psychodrama in America and this was reflected in the emphasis coming from the Hoewell training course and others that followed in its wake. Nevertheless, outright conflict has been avoided and psychodrama has found a sympathetic response from some psychotherapists trained in a psychoanalytic mode, including myself.

It should be understood, however, that this book is an account of my experience and training as a psychodramatist, in the first instance, and the manner in which I have been influenced by certain central analytic concepts. It is not the work of a psychoanalyst working through psychodrama, and no prior knowledge of psychoanalytic concepts on the part of the reader is required.

This book is written to encourage trainees in psychodrama and psychotherapy and counselling to look closely and with understanding at the manner in which these disparate approaches to human mental health can work together. Much can be gained if rivalrous conflict is avoided and respect is offered for the creative possibilities of different approaches, sometimes working separately, sometimes together. Freudians do not possess psychoanalysis and followers of Moreno do not possess psychodrama. Rogers would certainly never wish to be seen as having exclusive rights to person-centred counselling theory, although he might be disappointed at the relatively slow development of counselling client groups in this country and the individualization of much of the work offered to clients.

This book will, I hope, appeal to all those working in the world of mental health who look for creative approaches to alleviating the distress of mental and emotional suffering. The text guides readers through the main ideas, and the structure and techniques of psychodrama, and illustrates its method and effects through the discussion of vignettes, which are used for illustrative purposes. These will be drawn from my experience as a psychodrama trainee/trainer and practitioner of some 20 years' standing.

As I write a wonderful natural phenomenon has taken place in the form of a magnificent psychodrama for many people: the death and rebirth of the sun through a full eclipse. Those witnessing it in Cornwall, Devon and the Channel Islands spoke with feelings of awe and wonder at the experience shared, not only as a scientific wonder, but as a metaphorical statement concerning our universal vulnerability as human beings.

I hope this book will interest not only enthusiasts and those who are already convinced of the merits of psychodrama but also those who are unaware or even sceptical of the value of psychodrama as psychotherapy. I hope, too, that the book is written in a style that will make it readable to ordinary members of the public who simply wish to know out of a spirit of human enquiry.

A number of books have been published mainly concerned with the techniques of psychodrama, advocating its usefulness. Moreno himself wrote at great length to this end. Mostly these books address practitioners and trainees in psychodrama and are relatively conventional in the sense that they are primarily concerned with Moreno's theories of role, drama and catharsis. While being concerned with the same ideas, this book attempts to place psychodrama within the context of a growing interest in both individual and group analysis, the importance of the unconscious as well as the conscious in the conduct of our affairs, and finally the significance of the relationship between therapist and client in the process of therapy whether it be in the individual consultation or in the setting of the therapy group.

Don Feasey
October 2000

Introduction

I write as a psychodramatist who has found certain insights from the world of psychoanalysis useful – especially those derived from the founder of it all, Sigmund Freud. I am not assuming the position of a psychoanalyst in this text although I acknowledge my debt to that influence. First and foremost the book is written from my experience as a psychodramatist and it is intended to advance the value of that therapy to those already experienced in its theory and practice and to those who are making tentative approaches in that direction.

Good Practice in Psychodrama has been written to explore the theory and practice of psychodrama in a way that will interest psychotherapists in training, experienced practitioners in psychodrama, and therapists from other therapeutic disciplines who are curious and who see possibilities in psychodrama for their own preferred ways of working.

The book is based on my own work as a psychoanalytic psychotherapist, dramatherapist and psychodramatist for some 20 years. The illustrations and vignettes are drawn from practitioner experience both in private clinical practice and training and in work within the NHS. I have taken obvious steps to protect the identity of the clients concerned.

In that respect it is a personal account. It describes my own approach to psychodrama practice whilst recognizing that there are other psychodramatists who might approach the work from other directions and with a different emphasis. Indeed it is my recognition of the manner in which what might be described as 'classical' Moreno psychodrama was being influenced by varying and developing schools of thought from the world of psychotherapy (Holmes, 1992; Wilkins, 1999) that, in part, motivated this book.

Good Practice in Psychodrama introduces an analytical perspective. Throughout the book I use the terms 'psychodynamic', 'analytic' and 'psychoanalytic' synonymously. There are, of course, a number of schools of psychoanalysis that, to some extent, contend with each other, using different language and employing different emphases. Despite differences in theoretical positions, all the present schools of psychoanalysis accept the basic concepts that I introduce in this book, which are fundamental to psychoanalytic psychotherapy. The book lays an emphasis upon the presence and nature of the unconscious and the importance of what is known as 'transference', especially within the context of the dynamics of interpersonal relationships. These experiences are not limited to the world of psychoanalytic theory or experience – on the contrary, they occur in everyday life and many people recognize the existence of an unconscious life and also acknowledge how they are affected by transferential relationships. How often we have overheard the expression 'she treats me like her mother' (spoken approvingly or disapprovingly) as part of a conversation in the bread shop while waiting to pick up a loaf. The experience is commonplace.

The book is limited to an examination of the manner in which a psychodramatist may use an understanding and acceptance of the importance of *some* basic psychoanalytical assumptions in the practice of psychodrama as a therapeutic or training process. It is written from the point of view of a psychodramatist who has found these analytical concepts, drawn from both individual and group work, very useful in the process of therapeutic work. It is *not* written from the point of view of a psychoanalyst working through psychodrama.

The reader does not need much knowledge of psychoanalytical theory in all its variations. A lay person's familiarity will prove sufficient. Neither should the lay person be deterred by his or her lack of practical experience of psychodrama. It will not matter, either, if such a person has not read a word of Moreno, its inventor and founder. All the necessary vocabulary of psychodrama is explained.

Psychodrama is a multifarious way of working with people in a number of experiential situations. The content and technique of psychodrama is easily applied to learning situations. As a former trainer I used its methods to help staff groups learn about the dynamics of their social relationships within a work context. I used it to help community nurses learn simple methods of counselling within the context of their visits to private homes. I used it within the context of a youth theatre project that I was leading, to help the adolescent members manage their personal processes of emotional learning. I used it in my work as a teacher and youth worker trainer.

This book is deliberately restricted to the world of therapy. Having said that, I know that discerning readers will see other possibilities for using its method. My illustrations are all drawn from the world of therapy, and it is my aim to influence the world of mental health, enabling psychodrama to become a more accepted and developed way of working with clients, both in the public and private health sectors.

Perhaps the most important quality of psychodrama is its insistence on the notion of spontaneity as a highly valued human attribute. When present in the psychodrama performance spontaneity is a good guide to the essence of healthy human experience. I liken it to 'free association' when the client in psychoanalytical therapy is invited to speculate and explore the world of feeling and action in an unrestricted, non-judgemental way. In this respect the therapies come close together, demonstrating an essential respect for the client and the client's right to take a powerful and determining role in his or her own therapy, often in stark contrast to the medical mental health model.

In the interest of the wellbeing of former trainees, clients and patients, all names, places and times of psychodrama enactments described in this book have been altered to secure as high as degree of confidentiality as possible. Sometimes the gender of participants has been altered to help preserve anonymity.

Until recent years it was assumed that the fictional protagonist in any textbook would probably be male and would be referred to throughout a text as 'he'. I have decided to change the gender and choose the fictional figure to be a female who is referred to throughout as 'she' or 'her'.

This is partly an act to redress the balance of convention towards women and also as a mark of respect I feel for those pioneers of psychodrama whom I have known who are women, especially Doreen Elefthery, my trainer and supervisor.

Don Feasey

CHAPTER 1

Historical overview

> 'Now is the winter of our discontent
> Made glorious summer'
>
> Shakespeare. *The Tragedy of King Richard the Third.* Act 1, Scene 1.

The curtain opens

Scene 1 – prologue

An NHS hospital in the north of England. The psychotherapy clinic. A summer afternoon.

The whole community that day was assembled in the large group-therapy space when Janet and I made our way along the corridor and into the room. We paused at the door. The group was sitting in a large circle. Everyone was watching us. My chair and the co-therapy chair were empty. The patients, about 25 of them, watched us expectantly. Sitting among them were a number of staff, group therapists of different persuasions. They watched us too. Joan, the psychiatrist, was sitting with her usual nervous, tense smile. The smile was not for us. It was rather an inwardly directed smile. She was waiting for the protagonist to appear. The atmosphere was rich with expectations.

Janet sat down first. I followed her and took my seat. A deep silence pervaded the room. Now eyes looked away from us. Only a covert glance or two came in my direction. I sat silently too. I was quite well aware that Edmond, the chosen and named protagonist of that day, was not present. So was everyone else. They were all waiting to see how I would respond. The group analyst in me counselled me to sit still and wait for the community to respond verbally, but already the body language was fluent. Edmond's absence challenged the culture of the community and the planned psychotherapy session.

A few minutes dragged by. The silence was becoming oppressive. New members of the community were finding it hard to bear the tension of waiting. I expected one of them to speak. Then suddenly, Mary, a young woman new to the community, in her second week, lifted her head and addressed Janet. Her voice was lost for, as she spoke, a great sigh of murmuring spread around the group, there was a rustling of bodies and a squeak of moving seats as a figure began to push among them looking for a place to sit down. It was Edmond, of course. Red of face, untidy in appearance, defiant in posture, he finally found a seat and joined the group. The psychodrama had started.

This account places psychodrama as an important therapy within the life of a day therapeutic community. It shares the same integrity and value as large- and small-group analysis, art therapy, dramatherapy and relaxation sessions within the weekly programme of community life. The session described above is a remembered account from some 10 years ago. Psychodrama was not regarded as a novelty or some fringe therapy – an exotic afterthought to the life of the therapeutic community; rather, it was trusted and valued by everyone, patients and staff alike, for the part it played in community life. It should be remembered that as long ago as 1943 Foulkes – one of the few psychiatrists of the time to have knowledge of Moreno (Foulkes, 1948) – came to work at Northfield Hospital and brought psychodrama with him. It would be foolish to deny that in our community it was special. I was the only trained psychodramatist in the staff group at the time, although many of the staff were very interested in the technique.

Although closely related to psychodrama, dramatherapy has its own special culture and history of development as a psychotherapy, especially in the UK. A number of dramatherapists are skilled in the practice of psychodrama, moving easily between the techniques of both. Reference to dramatherapy and its literature will be found in Chapter 14.

Drama, in the form of theatre, has always found a deeply valued place in the social life of human beings. It is known that the Ancient Greeks believed that the enactment of their powerful didactic tragedies purified their communities and was a powerful therapeutic experience for actors and audience alike (Nicoll, 1955). In our own time to watch a modern day audience deeply attentive to an Arthur Miller drama, such as *Death of a Salesman* or *All my Sons*, is to witness a large group of people experiencing a catharsis through identification with the characters depicted on stage, sharing their personal and universal tragic experience at an emotional level. Alternatively, an audience rocking with laughter, as in a recent production of Noel Coward's *Nude with a Violin* at the Royal

Exchange Theatre, Manchester, demonstrates the profound need we all have to mock foolish pretentiousness and to celebrate the common frail humanity we all equally share. The same theme was explored tragically by the actor Tom Courtney in a magnificent production of Shakespeare's *King Lear* at the same theatre. What could be more cleansing and therapeutic in the broad meaning of that word? Bertolt Brecht (1998) speaks feelingly of the way that ordinary working people dramatize their lives, especially their conflicts and victories. Almost in spite of his orthodox Marxist background, he pays respect to the therapeutic energy of the dramatic experience. He notes how the recall of experience and its dramatic retelling in role – for example 'he said' and 'I said', all coloured with tone of voice, inflection and volume and amplified with gesture and body posture – confirms the experience and places it in an analytical position from which it can be viewed and assessed. A typical disputation Brechtian role play ends with 'Well, I tell you, after that little up and downer he won't come the old acid with me again, he will get his bloody rent on time and keep out of my hair!' Victory is celebrated but the realism of the social balance is acknowledged in the simple line 'he will get his bloody rent on time'.

In the contemporary scene, the phenomenon of the TV soap opera is ubiquitous. The small dramas of everyday life daily command attentive and loyal audiences who seem absolutely entranced by the dramatized social, domestic and working lives of the characters concerned. For many of the TV watchers it appears that the characters depicted are 'real'.

Back in the 1950s, studying drama at Trent Park College with the late Jim Burton (1955), I was a young married man with two children. I worked part time in a London East End play centre to earn a little money to pay the rent and the gas bill. This was in the days when, as a society, we were not ashamed of spending public money on the care and entertainment of our children. The London County Council was a good provider. We had an open day when parents, play workers, councillors and officials came to have a look at us. I was asked to run an open drama workshop with the children, which I did. As usual, I got out the dressing-up box and talked to them about what was required. They listened politely then proceeded to play their usual drama. Jane was mother, bossy, quick to temper, very active and free with her cuffs and slaps. Jenny was the cheeky daughter who 'gave lip'. Jimmy was the tearaway ten-year-old son, leader of a gang, proud of it but respectful to his mum and careful of his father's wrath. Bill, the oldest boy, about 14 years old, was dad. Coming home tired from work he flopped in a chair and required to be waited on hand and foot by his daughter. But he was careful not to 'mouth' his wife. He barked out a few orders to his son. Other children played variations on these roles as friends and neighbours. In all about 20 of them took part.

There was no shape to the drama. No great contrived climax. It just went on and on. The only controversial figure was an older girl who played Miss Smith from the 'Social', a feared and despised figure. Mother, sisters and brothers, neighbours and friends, all sat entranced and watched with rapt attention until I brought it summarily to an end.

This explains, in some part, why we cherish the drama and our playwrights in our oral history even if we only reward them sparsely with money and social status. And as for actors – they remain today, as they have always been, adored on the stage as they depict our follies, triumphs and despairs, but not entirely trusted off stage. Perhaps we fear and envy the magic of their performances. One successful film was *Shakespeare in Love* where the ordinariness and genius of Shakespeare, the man, was celebrated along with the humour, sadness and beauty of his plays. The film was particularly British in its appeal. Cinema audiences could be heard murmuring quietly to themselves whole chunks of Shakespearean speech as they recognized them in the dialogue of the film. Audiences were delighted as they recognized the 'in' jokes in the film drawn from the Elizabethan and Jacobean repertoire of plays first performed over 300 years ago. Embodied in the collective conscious and unconscious of the population are whole segments of the lives of Shakespearean characters from a host of plays. At some time or another we are all Hamlet, Macbeth, Richard II or III, Henry IV and V, Romeo and Juliet, Ophelia, Lady Macbeth, Hamlet's mother, Lear's daughters, Gonerill, Regan, Cordelia and so on; the list is endless. From time to time these are acknowledged, but most of the time they remain below the level of immediate consciousness, working away as emotional and intellectual influences of barely acknowledged significance.

Actors play characters, take on roles. And so do all the rest of us. To quote Act 2, Scene 7 of Shakespeare's *As You Like It:* 'All the world's a stage/And all the men and women merely players.'

Moreno, the inventor of psychodrama, did not invent the notion of 'role' although he had plenty to say about it. Without reading a word of Moreno (1934) most of us could identify the roles we play through the drama of our lives, our loves and hates, achievements and failures, within which there are frequently highly specific roles that we perform with consummate skill: husbands, wives, partners, fathers, mothers, sons, daughters, grandparents, uncles, aunts, cousins, nephews, nieces, neighbours, best friends, acquaintances, workers, employees, employers, landlords, tenants and so forth. In fact it is this ability to play varying roles with sincerity and conviction that delineates us as healthy human beings. It is quite obvious that those afflicted with pathological neuroses or who are mentally ill, in the psychiatric sense of the word, are really quite incapable of the flexibility and sensitivity required to play demanding roles.

Moreno's genius was to recognize this and formulate a therapy that, through dramatization, helped to restore the skill of healthy role playing. The technique, which will be described in some detail later in this book, enabled the performers to enter into fundamental human roles, explore them, evaluate them and gain insight and psychic strength in the process. I think Foulkes would have been interested in this work because Moreno, in the first instance, placed drama into the context of group psychotherapy. It is true that it is possible to work psychodramatically with an individual the usual and orthodox setting is the group. However, before exploring this any further, I am reminded of an occasion when a male client, of some standing, in an individual therapy session, tears pricking his eyes, suddenly moved into dramatic mode. His voice rose to a near falsetto. His head lifted, his shoulders tightened up and his fingers stiffened as he began to speak:

Scene 2

'Don't be such a cry baby John, stand up, stop rolling about on the grass, you will mess up your clothes. What a state you are in. Stop crying for goodness sake, big boys don't cry. You are behaving just like a silly little girl; except your sister would never make such a fuss. I hope you don't behave like this at the infant school. Goodness knows what your father would think of you if he could see you. Now go straight indoors, wash your face, tidy yourself up and don't come back until you are prepared to be more sensible and stop making a fuss.'

All this dialogue poured out of him quite spontaneously and I listened in silence, attentively. There was a pause. He looked at me. 'That was my mother.'

I looked at him and said 'Yes, her voice, exactly as you remember it, I should think.' He nodded. He began to rub the tears away. I said 'Well I suppose you are telling me your mother found it very difficult to cope with feelings of pain and distress, especially tears, especially your tears.'

From time to time the psychoanalytical psychotherapist or counsellor witnesses such an 'acted out memory'. It is commonplace in our own private experience of ourselves to hear the voice of, perhaps, a dead mother or father speaking to us sometimes in tones of affection, encouragement, remorse or admonishment. So it is not surprising that clients will remember and reproduce the voice from the past with remarkable faithfulness.

But it is exceptional rather than general for a psychodrama to be conducted with an individual. Generally speaking psychodrama is conducted in a group especially convened to work through psychodrama. Moreno seems not to have paid much attention to the unconscious life of the group; rather, he took a sociometric approach to group life and his most important and earliest study in America was based on his work with delinquent girls at the Hudson School for Girls and at Sing Sing Prison. In both institutions his aim was for a more liberal and essentially community-based form of social treatment for the inmates. He constructed questionnaires to ascertain individual preferences for friendship choice among the inmates, hoping always to tease out the factors that would throw insight into the deviant behaviour and possible social therapeutic responses. This interactionist approach has been reflected and built upon in more recent times by the American advocates of social group work theory and by Joan Matthews, formerly a lecturer at the National College for Training Youth Leaders in Leicester, who published *Working with Youth Groups* (Matthews, 1966). Another lecturer from the National College, Bernard Davies, produced another book *The Use of Groups in Social Work Practice* (Davies, 1975), which addressed similar concerns from a social work perspective. This book provides a useful bibliography of group work writing, largely based on social group work theory. In 1972 I was privileged to take part in the BBC television series *Working with Youth 1972* and to contribute to the book of the series (Davies, 1975) where basic principles of group work approaches to the healthy development of young people were discussed, explained and evaluated. Although the approach is basically interactionist, implicit in much of the material is a concern with the unconscious communications of adolescent boys and girls.

The achievement of Moreno at constructing theories of group behaviour as early as the 1920s and 1930s has largely been lost. Possibly his own later preoccupation with psychodrama and his tendency to enter into conflict with those, like Slavson, whom he saw as rivals, removed him from the current list of distinguished group work theorists. But in this book it is his creative skill as the first psychodramatist that will be addressed, although a contemporary reading of group work would certainly contain an emphasis upon the unconscious life of groups and a number of psychodramatists today, including myself, acknowledge the need to take into account this phenomenon when working therapeutically.

This is not a book about psychoanalysis, but it would be impossible to develop its ideas without paying attention to the work of Freud and his successors. Freud was a contemporary of Moreno and upstaged him for attention both in Europe and in America, much to Moreno's chagrin.

Indeed, Moreno openly attacked and belittled Freud, who did not respond in a like manner.

Scene 3

Moreno met Freud briefly in 1914 and there was a brief exchange with Freud after Freud had delivered a lecture in the Vienna University Clinic of Psychiatry. Freud asked Moreno what he was doing. Freud had just delivered a lecture on dreams. 'Well', responded Moreno, 'you meet people in the artificial setting of your office. I meet them on the street and in their homes, in their natural surroundings. You analyse their dreams. I try to give them courage to dream again. I teach people how to play God . . . Freud looked at me as if puzzled, and smiled' (Moreno, 1964).

It was Moreno's misfortune that he was a contemporary of Freud and found Freud's position virtually unchallengeable when he moved to America in 1925. Whatever the virtue of their different therapeutic theories, it is a fact that Freud was embraced by very senior medical opinion in America – indeed, a far more influential group than the one in England led by Ernest Jones. Moreno had no such support when he came to America and his apparent need for conflict tended to leave him isolated and ignored by the psychiatric establishment. Later doctors such as the late Dean Elefthery, a distinguished psychiatrist/psychodramatist, together with his wife Doreen and Zerka Moreno, Moreno's second wife, did much to redress this situation and should be credited with advancing the 'cause' of psychodrama within American circles with a high degree of success. As a result of the early pioneering efforts by Moreno and his supportive contemporaries, the American Society for Group Psychotherapy and Psychodrama came into being and flourishes to this day.

As far as this book is concerned, what is being acknowledged and drawn from the psychoanalytic culture, is the influence of the unconscious in human affairs and the centrality of human psychological interaction and intra-action within the mind in the formation of a personality. As far as therapy goes, contemporary psychodramatists are paying close attention to the idea of 'transference' in as much as it plays an active psychological role in relationships. This applies to clients working in groups who experience transference relationships between each other and also, most importantly, towards the group conductor/s. As Yalom (1975) states, it is not a matter of whether transference exists – the issue is what do you do about it. Williams (1989) discusses and summarizes the current psychoanalytic views concerning the unconscious life of a therapy group and its application to the role of the leader in transference terms. He seems to acknowledge some force in the psychoanalytic position, especially as set out by

Foulkes (1948), but insists upon a multiplicity of group affects that sit in equal importance to that of leader-centred transference issues, normally advanced by group analytic analysts. It is obvious, however, that such psychoanalytical notions as: resistance, projective identification, denial, flight into either health or illness, free association and interpretation, regression and repression and symbolic behaviour may all be useful parts of the psychodramatist's repertoire of understanding in working through psychodrama. It is true that many contemporary trainers in psychodrama do not embrace this view, but such a perspective is not limiting if considered sensitively within the context of the actual client and the psychodramatic performance.

Scene 4

Mary never missed a psychodrama session. She would sit in the group, alert, attentive and apparently concerned. For weeks this was her position and disposition. When the moment of moving from group warm-up to protagonist identification came Mary would swiftly leave her chair, go across to the door of the room that lead out into the corridor and slip smoothly onto the carpet, her legs tucked under skirt, her back against the door. Her facial expression hardly changed. Her eyes stayed upon the psychodramatist with the same intense attention of interest. The group, accustomed to her manner, ignored her behaviour. She had a reputation for 'flight' from therapy groups and was often to be found in the community kitchen drinking coffee having slipped out of her therapy group. But she did not leave the psychodrama group room and always stayed for the closure.

The psychodramatist observed this behaviour and inhibited himself from direct confrontation at the time of Mary's gesture, her dramatic removal from the participating circle. However, he never failed to address the behaviour during the closure and Mary listened with rapt attention to his voice as he talked about her, albeit in the briefest of terms, interpreting her gesture rather than criticizing it, sometimes giving attention to her position as doorkeeper, 'in charge' of keeping the group together in the room and obstructing intruders. He was confident her time would come. He was also acutely aware of Mary's attachment to him and her desire not to share him with the rest of the group. Hence her disassociation from them and her intense eye contact with his figure.

In this scene, recalled from my years in the community group, I am drawing attention to the presence of transference (Kellermann, 1992) a topic that needs to be addressed in the common, universal language of psychotherapy. It has a many-layered presence in the psychodrama group as it is directed towards both client members and the director. As Yalom says, the issue is how to address it. A recipe cannot be given. On the contrary, the director has to analyse the process of the group (Williams, 1989) in relation to the individual members, the group as a whole, and the director himself, and then must try to reach an understanding of its meaning. Then the director acts. Psychodrama directors do this all the time, on their feet, as the process takes place. It does not seem to me that an appreciation of unconscious communication would impede understanding. On the contrary, what is often puzzling and confusing behaviour in the group becomes clear if the psychodramatist understands the presence of the unconscious in the life of the protagonist and how it may manifest itself in the psychodrama group.

Martineau (1989) draws attention to the fruitless conflicts that pursued, and were embraced by, Moreno during his life in America. Freud more-or-less ignored him, despite regular attacks upon psychoanalysis by Moreno, but others were drawn into the fray. Martineau wonders how much better Moreno might have fared if he had not allowed himself, as he said, 'to be the controversy'. How much less antagonism there might have been from other schools of therapeutic thought and how much more acknowledgement he would have received from his peers during his professional lifetime. I will resist an interpretation. Robin Skynner (1974) acknowledges Moreno's contribution to group therapy but reflects that Moreno impaired his own influence by 'developing a private language, rejecting past sources and ignoring other current developments'.

Nevertheless, Moreno has, somewhat surprisingly, emerged as a creative therapeutic force in Britain today and it seems that now is the time for a revaluation of his work and ideas, in a climate of tolerance, acceptance and discovery. It is this discovery and revival that is examined and explained in this book and, in the next chapter, we shall be looking at psychodrama and its place in the group psychotherapies in the UK today.

Chapter 2

Psychodrama is group psychotherapy

'The web of our life is of mingled yarn, good and ill together.'

Shakespeare. *All's Well that Ends Well.* Act 4. Scene 3.

'Some otherwise analytically oriented colleagues find psychodrama useful and practise it. I do not doubt that acting or role playing are valuable means of communication; this however, is very different from an analytical approach. If confined to the session and to the group as a whole, and with the sanction and even on the suggestion of the therapist, it is a different matter. The question is whether it is really necessary.'

Foulkes (1975)

For this psychotherapist, the answer to Foulkes is a resounding 'yes'. My training as a psychoanalytic psychotherapist took place individually and in groups and so did my training as a psychodramatist. In both cases the groups were closed groups with a consistent membership respecting the ethics of confidentiality and trust. The groups met over a lengthy period of time. The analytic group met for four years and the psychodrama group met for slightly longer, but less frequently. The supervision of my psychodramatic work took place in a group as well, but it was not closed and the membership varied considerably. The supervision also took place over a number of years.

For the purposes of this chapter I shall be discussing the nature of group psychotherapy and its relationship to psychodrama in the group. Looking back at these group experiences now, from a distance, certain questions arise. In the case of the group analytic experience there was no ambiguity concerning the nature of the group. It was a training therapy group and it was conducted by a training analyst in the manner of a psychoanalytic group experience. In the case of the psychodrama training group the nature of the group is more difficult to describe. How did it work? Was it like my client group? How far did my performance either as the protagonist, alter ego, group member, trainee director or co-director, relate to the group as a whole and my place in it?

Sue Jennings (1983) states quite firmly: 'with psychodrama no attention is paid to group process or dynamics. Sue is quite wrong in her observation. As a former client member of a number of psychodrama groups and director of even more, that was not my experience at all. The protagonist is in a *group* and will both consciously or unconsciously use the group experience in performance. Certainly, as a client, I was very aware of the group and my membership of it, including my 'place' in it, which changed from time to time.

Not so many years ago, in the group analytic movement, analysts would distinguish between (1) psychoanalysis of the individual in the group, (2) the psychoanalysis of the individual in her relationships in the group, (3) the psychoanalysis of the group itself, as a whole, especially in relation to the analyst. Fine hair splitting! Much resulting confusion.

I think that now group analysts would be less concerned with maintaining a 'pure' position, whatever it might be, and move dynamically with the needs of the individuals and the group through different emphases and perspectives, the limitation being in the confidence and ability of the therapist to vary and control shift in analytic stance and mode. That is probably true of psychodrama directors too. One may stick very firmly to the performance of the *individual* in the group and avoid concern for the psychological material of the *group as a whole*. Another director may be willing to confront or address, at a proper moment, the effect of the individual performance on the relationships within the group itself. Another director might notice the frequency of bids made by an individual to perform, using that perception to open up discussion of the situation and the group's response to it. A director might be very aware of reluctance to perform by a particular member, bringing it to the attention of the group. On the other hand the 'please sir, me sir' phenomenon might be evident and call for comment by the director or members of the group. Sometimes there may be a need to look at the use of alter ego figures – at *who* is chosen to perform *what* role, or perhaps to draw attention to the *frequency* or *absence* of doubling. Here I am suggesting that the process of the group provides rich therapeutic material.

Doubling is the process where one group member speaks for the protagonist, giving voice to possible thoughts and feelings.

Scene 5

Three professional women in a psychodrama training group in quick succession cast the same man drawn from the group as a major sexual figure in their life. He is described as dominant, bullying, demanding, insensitive and 'macho' in his attitudes to them. Although he was quite able to play these roles with dramatic conviction, supported with helpful doubling, nevertheless at the third time of casting he confessed in the closure to unease at the manner of the casting and the role he had been called upon to play each time. He confessed to jealousy towards other men in the group who were given more sympathetic roles to play in the psychodramas of the women protagonists. He posed certain concerns:

He felt the casting was too near the bone to his own problems with authority and his struggle with dominant women, especially those in caring professions . . . 'You know those bloody nurses who boss you around, make you feel like a five year old!'

He said 'I feel that in these roles I am playing, I am being asked to compete in a macho way with the younger men in the group. I have trouble with that anyway.' Some of the other men grinned sympathetically. 'I'm worried too', he went on 'that something in me is attracting these projections from the women in the group. I feel my natural masculinity is under attack. It also makes me wonder, what is it, in me, that I play these persecutory roles so well. I feel I am being repeatedly stereotyped and I want some help to break out of it from the group, especially the women. I'm fed up with playing "bad men".'

Virtually all this statement was aimed at the director in the closure of the group. A director has a choice about how to handle it. Some might see it entirely as an individual personal problem relating closely to issues of mothering and control in his childhood and the emerging oedipal struggle. Others, like myself, might feel it was a statement of importance to the group as a whole, conveyed through me and my place as the leader of a group. In transference terms he was challenging me to be a caring, sensitive authority figure, enabling and releasing him, perhaps in contrast to other experience in his life. Kellerman (1992) outlines what may be regarded as a commonly accepted definition of the term drawn from the work of Freud as early as 1905.

Kellerman (1992) describes it in the following terms: 'The patient comprehends the therapist in a manner which is unrealistic and coloured by the significant figures in the patient's life. Attitudes and feelings which are "advanced" to the present, but which correspond to the patient's past, are brought forth through what the patient says (to the therapist).'

This phenomenon will be discussed throughout this book along with Moreno's notion of *tele*, which, in contrast to *transference*, is the word used to describe a *real* relationship between client and therapist, which is vested in mutual regard and concern. In other words it is not a mere fantasy activated by projection; rather, it is substantiated and facilitated by the quality of the relationship as it is experienced between the psychodramatist and client.

Obviously, there can be no definitive answer to the dilemma posed by this particular patient as described by Kellerman. The context determines the response of the director and especially her knowledge of the speaker; what has gone before in the life of the psychodrama group is often of great importance. It is clear that the notion of the psychodrama group as being without a significant transference process is challenged when such an incident takes place. In the instance quoted here the client was being held by the group in a position from which he was constantly trying to emerge – perhaps from the victim of the controlling mother or inadequate father who failed to support his earlier struggles for independence. Very frustrating.

Scene 6

A woman patient in a hospital psychodrama group is in a role-reversal situation with her former husband. She is being constantly 'doubled' by another woman patient who speaks with almost uncontrollable anger, distress, complaint and suffering. The protagonist says 'Well yeah he is a bit of a shit, but not that bad. I don't feel so oppressed by him, I tried to stand up for myself. He thought I was a real shrew!'

On completion of her doubling to the protagonist the patient found it difficult to leave the scene, or leave the protagonist and go back to her seat in the group.

As Dean Elefthery (late director of the International Foundation of Human Relations) might have said: 'whose psychodrama is this anyway?' The director, in such circumstances, has to *protect* the protagonist from too much doubling, too many projections. At the same time she has to note with concern the *need* of the group member, doubling in such a forceful manner. She has to find time and space to deal with issues raised, sometimes in the period that is called 'sharing' that which comes before the closure of the group. Or it might take the form of a new psychodrama where the member doubling now becomes the protagonist.

Scene 7

A young woman complains bitterly about her mother's failure to prepare her for menstruation. 'God what a bloody, yes that's the right word, bloody shock it was, when I began to bleed. I couldn't say a thing to her. I talked to Sal, my friend Sal, she knew what I had to do. I felt so dirty, blood coming from down there.' Jane another group member joins in.

'You know, you only ever talk about sex when Jim comes to run a psychodrama group with us. Otherwise you avoid the subject like the plague. I wonder what that's all about?' Uncomfortable silence.

Here a direct reference is being made to the director in the group and the presence of an important dynamic for two of the women concerned, who notice how his presence appears to affect the concerns of individual group members. In this instance it is the issue of sexuality. And the director mentioned is male. Suddenly a new issue is on the group agenda. How should it be handled? It does not lie in my power to give the answer at this moment but the issue is raised and should not be ignored. What is obvious is that gender, sexual life and censorship are emerging as issues. This may or may not be something the director feels he can cope with when suddenly his presence becomes a subject of speculation. I can recall a particularly painful episode for myself when directing a hospital psychodrama group.

Scene 8

A man in the group proposes himself for a psychodrama. He wishes to look at his past, the time of the Korean War where he tortured and murdered prisoners in his charge. All this was known to the authorities above him and covertly approved of. As he spoke I was monitoring my feelings, feeling panicky and faint. Actual sadism is a subject I find increasingly hard to bear. I have vivid war memories of the reporting of concentration camp atrocities – horrific photos of public executions and torture. I visited Belsen, a scene of mass graves, a notorious starvation death camp in the British Zone of Germany, shortly after the end of World War Two. I also have powerful memories of infancy, hospitalized, when I felt persecuted and abandoned, sometimes treatment procedures experienced as sadistic attacks, painful and frightening. I knew I was not safe enough to work with this patient. The group seemed to pick it up. Unconscious communication, perhaps. They were being distant toward the proposal, not supporting the would-be protagonist. They were looking to me for guidance. My co-therapist, a woman psychologist, picked up my hesitation, the barely concealed distress. She knew me well as a therapist and moved the group on to look at other proposals. I felt immensely relieved. This was discussed during the peer supervision meeting between the therapy team after the closure of the group.

In this example I am showing that, as the director of the group, I am vulnerable to group interactions – to the group process. Rather than denying the process or simply trying to bluff my way through it, my choice was to acknowledge its force and use the understanding of the co-therapist and the disposition of the group to resolve the matter. The reader should note at this juncture that this was not an example of counter-transference to the patient by me; these feelings were not coming from my unconscious in an unrecognizable form. Quite the contrary – I was aware of the source and power of the feelings from the moment they became manifest. As Kellerman (1979) wrote, the counter-transference experience arises from the unconscious in a much more disguised and distorting manner and is that much more difficult to identify and deal with.

In this instance we came back to the incident at the time of closure and during debriefing with my co-therapist. This included dealing with the distress of the patient who found his proposal refused by the group. All these scenes relating to the nature of group life are taken from my years of working in a day therapeutic community. Set in a hospital, the patients followed a 12-week, daily programme of group psychotherapy that included psychodrama on a weekly basis. Small analytic groups took place every day and there were daily large-group and community meetings; a thoroughgoing regime. The experience of the psychodrama group could and did enter the small and large analytic groups and was referred to quite openly in these settings.

In my own psychodrama training the group was closed. This ensured a very stable membership and when anyone left, which only happened rarely, he or she was not replaced. In the hospital it was different. The group was stable, but it was a slow, open, permanent group, admitting new members as patients left. This made for a somewhat different culture. Mostly it was signified by 'old' members of the group introducing new members to the culture and, as a result, there was a pecking order of experience and seniority, which had to be taken into account by the director. It was virtually an imperative for the director to note group process and to work in response to his understanding of what was taking place.

In the article mentioned earlier by Jennings (1973), she identified the following human experiences as the curative factors in psychodrama: empathy, identification and participation. I take it for granted that she includes catharsis. Both Freud in the early days and Moreno placed emphasis on catharsis as an important feature of therapy. We should remember that Freud was, in his early stages of development as a psychoanalyst, heavily influenced by the hypnotherapeutic dramas he witnessed in Paris, conducted by the then leading French psychiatrist Charcot. Much emphasis was placed in Paris on catharsis, which impressed Freud, although he had difficulty in reproducing the same effects in his own work when he returned to Vienna. At the time neurotic disorder was often labelled as 'hysteria'. This often took the form of the conversion of emotional states, 'affects', into physical demonstrations and defects. These hysterical conversions are not as common today, although many patients complain of physical disorders that doctors find difficult to diagnose and treat with formal medical interventions. Among these are back troubles, aches and pains in body and limbs, headaches and migraines, fatigue, stomach disturbances, mysterious comings and goings of what are labelled viral infections, sleep disorder, allergies of all kinds. The list is pretty well endless. I find that it is commonplace for a client, coming for therapy, to complain of physical problems for a short while and then apparently she loses interest in them and they receive very little attention in the therapeutic conversation.

The last case of hysterical paralysis I saw was in Poland about 12 years ago.

Scene 9

Rastow is a rural residential therapeutic community just outside of Warsaw. A community meeting was in progress in the form of a psychodramatic conversation. A young man had completed a piece of work and a young woman, Magda, who could not stand or walk, had been listening to the conversation with intense interest and distress. She had been virtually carried into the group by other patients, although the therapeutic staff did not lend a hand. Throughout the exchanges she had kept a tight, fixed grimace on her face. She stared at me and clutched her stomach, pulling her knees close to her chest. As the young man poured scorn on women, his failure in sexual relationships always attributed to hopeless, rejecting women, Magda grew more and more distressed. Soon she began to weep noisily. The whole community became very quiet and still. No one interrupted her. She continued to stare at me, tears streaming down her face as if to dramatize and challenge my place in the large group. Suddenly the group conductor/psychodramatist, George, spoke to her and she nodded and began to try to stand. Another patient moved across the circle and stood in front of her. She listened intently to him. Her eyes were now downcast but she is speaking, clearly and coherently 'warming up' the young male patient with information about her former lover. Now the male patient in role began to answer her. She grew more excited and angry, her voice lifted. She made another effort to stand, nearly succeeded, but collapsed back into her chair. The young man, 'auxiliary ego', walked away from her and began to laugh scornfully, hissing out derogatory remarks to her and waving her away with his hands and arms. His tone and scorn were plain and evident.

Suddenly she made a heroic effort and with a great push with her hands against the arms of the chair she was on her feet, swaying, knees buckling, shouting at him. She stumbled towards him and at that point fell swooningly towards the floor. The community group watched all this impassively. A member on the group left her chair and went and stood beside the prone Magda and began speaking to and for her, doubling quietly and sympathetically, urging her to 'stand up' for herself, both physically and metaphorically. But she did not touch her. It took Magda another three attempts before she stood again, this time with the woman alter ego standing beside her. She swayed, her arm reached to the floor and momentarily saved herself from sinking to the floor. This was repeated several times. Her posture was of struggle and recovery. I expected her to fall but she retained her position of precarious balance. She began to speak to the male actor who turned to look at her, giving her his full attention. I felt a sense of relief pass through me and imagined it shared by the whole community. As the scene ended the feeling of pleasure and approval in the group at the success of Magda in overcoming her 'paralysis' was palpable.

Afterwards I spoke to George and pointed out her eye contact with me and her focus on my presence. He laughed at me and said: 'Well, Don, you were the heroic stranger, a godlike presence from England who was going to rescue her from her paralysis, everyone in the community is talking about you.' Then with a wicked grin 'I'm sure you are enjoying all this attention.'

Such catharsis is not all that common in the group situation. When it occurs it is usually very moving, affecting the feelings of the whole group membership. Often the expression is of intense sadness or grief accompanied by tears. Usually, but not always, the reaction of the group is affirmative and celebratory. The desired outcome is that the catharsis leads to a more balanced view of the protagonist's life enjoyed by her and the group. At these moments the group process takes on a powerful therapeutic presence as the catharsis is shared by the remaining members of the group. Moreno (1946) identifies the 'audience' – the group membership – as one of the five instruments of psychodrama. Apart from helping the protagonist in the performance of the drama he writes: 'the audience is helped by the subject, thus becoming the patient itself, the situation is reversed. The audience sees itself, that is one of its collective syndromes, portrayed on the stage.'

Apart from catharsis it is obvious that many other group factors play a part in the therapy of the group. To illustrate this I would point to Yalom (1975). He proposes a number of what he calls curative factors. Jennings (1983) talks about learning rather than cure, but her intention is clear enough: she is pointing to the therapeutic features of psychodrama. Yalom is identifying the same processes in group psychotherapy but his list is far longer and more specific than Jennings'. He identifies:

- instillation of hope;
- universality of experience;
- imparting of information;
- altruism;
- creative recapitulation of the primary family group;
- development of socializing techniques;
- imitative behaviour;
- interpersonal learning;
- group cohesiveness;
- catharsis;
- existential factors (coming to terms with everyday realities).

It seems quite obvious that these are present in the psychodrama group as potential curative factors, coming into emphasis from time to time, depending upon the specific circumstances of the psychodrama in its entirety. Moreno himself spoke of the significance of psychodrama as an interpersonal therapy 'a meeting of two; eye to eye, face to face' (quoted in Kellerman, 1992).

For anyone who has run a psychodrama group over a sustained period of time, it is obvious that some of these factors are operational from time to time. One of the problems for a number directors is that they often do not have this long-term experience and the groups they train in, or conduct, are more ephemeral and consequently less revealing of these positive features. Time is all important and the full therapeutic value of the experience only becomes clear in the long run.

Psychodrama as a therapy shares these factors of positive experience with other group therapies but also shares the negative aspect when the curative factors are reversed:

- shared despair;
- individuation of experience;
- secrecy, including pairing where a couple of members form an exclusive alliance;
- selfishness;
- pathological recapitulation of the primary family group in destructive activity;
- uncooperative hostility in social behaviour;
- acting out in hysterical flight behaviour – this often takes place outside group meetings;

- denial;
- intragroup rivalry, pairing, splitting and subgrouping;
- depression and withdrawal;
- paranoid projection to a hostile world.

Directors, performers and protagonists all know that when such conditions are found in the psychodrama group then the energy and creativity of the group is blocked and frustration prevails, inhibiting the therapy of the group.

It is rare for all these pathological features to surface at one time in a group but their potential is always present and is experienced from time to time by psychodrama directors in the course of their therapeutic work.

My view is that the psychodrama group is likely to be close in its essence, as against its techniques, to many other therapy groups. I shall be looking with more detail at the question of techniques later in the book but for the moment would suggest we give attention to the article written by Anthony Ryle (1976) who outlined certain necessary conditions attached to the idea of a therapy group.

He suggested a group of about eight, meeting regularly with a therapist for a fixed period of time, usually one-and-a-half hours. He took the place of the group for granted, but I would emphasize its importance. Security of tenure is a must for a psychodrama group, as well as sufficient space in which to work to meet the conditions of psychodramatic performance. As far as number is concerned, psychodrama can be very effective in groups much larger than eight and large closed psychodrama groups may be especially effective. This was probably true of the Polish example quoted earlier when about 20 people were present.

Ryle describes the phases of group development as follows:

- the anxious, mistrustful, ambivalent, dependent phase; the group is technically naive and inexperienced;
- the working phase: trusting, open, group-centred, working with and challenging leadership, family conscious, reflecting and creating experience, technically skilful with know how of psychotherapy language and activity;
- the phase of loss and gain as old members leave and new members arrive. The group temporarily regresses to phase one but behaves more confidently, tolerating loss and assimilating new blood.

What sometimes confuses these issues for trainee directors is that they attend weekend and ad hoc training groups where the conditions of group membership are not predictable or attached to regular attendance. This situation is, I am glad to say, changing as trainers become more aware of the value of a constant and predictable membership in regular attendance. But it was not always so. This is ironic when it is remembered that Moreno was one of the pioneers of an understanding of group life and dynamics. It is true that much of his work in sociometrics has been 'lost' through neglect and superseded by others in the field and his 'language' of sociometrics is now largely unused in academic circles, but his influence still resonates in modern psychodrama practice and Culpan (1979) writes:

> He [the director] should be knowledgeable of action techniques, effective in exploring the development and maintenance of affiliative relationships, and understand the dynamics of personal choice and its relationship to personal growth. Such training is not a matter of the therapist 'picking up' some more skills but rather the laying of a foundation for influencing his viewpoint of man. By viewing man as a social being, functioning in the context of others, one cannot possible perceive man as a solitary creature.

Every group has to deal with the issue of leadership. In the *training* psychodrama group the course trainer is the leader. Members may take it in turns to act as the pychodramatic director. In the psychodrama *therapy* group the designated leader is the director. She has a function that is laid down by the culture of the group, its customary practices, its formal rituals and roles. It is in strong contrast, apparently, to the stance of the analytic group leader or the Rogerian facilitator. This sometimes causes confusion to participants and directors in the world of psychodrama. Within the culture of group analysis there is a tradition of passive, interpretative leadership (Ezriel, 1952; Bion, 1959; Foulkes, 1975). This tradition stems from the work of Freud and his views on the subject of transference.

In 1959 there was a lively discussion of a number of psychoanalytic topics, the most important being that of the nature of transference, countertransference, interpersonal therapy, group psychotherapy and the nature and significance of the unconscious. Moreno (1946) writes: 'The time has come to evaluate the advances made by psychotherapy and to spell out, if possible, the common denominators of all its forms.' He continues: 'How can the various methods be brought into agreement, into a single comprehensive system?' It sometimes seems strange that contemporary psychodramatists and writers seem unhappy to engage in the same dialogue that Moreno himself faced and debated in a psychotherapeutic manner. Martineau's (1989) book outlines the range of this discussion and the range of experienced contemporary therapists who engaged with

Moreno in serious psychotherapeutic debate. Blatner (1973) discusses the affiliation of other psychotherapies to the psychodramatic method.

He quotes the instance of the Oedipal conflict, a central concern of Freudian psychoanalytic theory and comments on the manner in which the conflict emerges in the psychodramatic context. The following is a clear example from my own practice.

Scene 10 – An NHS day therapeutic community

The community has gathered to participate in the psychodrama of George, a 40-year-old bachelor who lives with his father and mother in a small terraced house in a rather depressed working-class district. George is nervous. He has seen several psychodramas whilst a patient in the community and made one or two tentative efforts at sharing with protagonists. He is a modest rather self-effacing man whose life has become more and more restricted and now suffers from agoraphobia, which leaves him virtually housebound with his elderly mother and father. Today he has volunteered to do a psychodrama. I am directing. We meet in an empty space, in a circle of patients and one co-therapist who sometimes works as a professional auxiliary. We have a relatively short discussion and decide jointly that it might be useful to have a talk with his parents and explore the dilemma of his phobia with them, using role reversal and doubling to help him get closer to the problem.

I ask him where the meeting should take place. He looks surprised. It appears to him there is only one place to meet – that is in the sitting room of the family home. I ask him first to describe the room and then to begin to assemble pieces of furniture to re-create the memory of the room tangibly. He has little difficulty in describing the room that he has inhabited with them for some 40 years. He starts to get the furniture organized. The furniture available to him in the psychodrama space is heavy and cumbersome. Far from ideal. I can see some members of the community are itching to help him, as he struggles with the weight and shape of the furniture, to get everything into place. But no one moves; everyone restrains a desire to 'help' George. First he places a waste paper bin in one corner of the 'stage' to represent the television set. There is a little joke about it being nothing but a load of rubbish. George grins apologetically and says to the audience 'I spend hours in front of the bloody thing.' There are sympathetic murmurs from the group. At last he has put everything in place. I ask him to look at the scene he has created carefully and see if it is 'right'. It is, to his satisfaction. I have already noticed a special feature of the set. He has only placed two chairs in front of the TV set. I press him again. 'Is that it George, are you sure there is nothing else you want to put into the scene?' He looks at it intently. 'Well there is usually a vase of flowers on the table.' He spots a plant in a pot in the psychodrama room, goes across and brings it to his scene, placing it carefully on the table. 'That's better' he remarks and looks pleased with himself.

I can feel a rising tension in the audience. Numbers of them are now aware of the missing third chair. Then Audrey rises quietly from her chair, glances at me, I give her a nod, and she moves into a position to double for George.

He is aware of her presence as she touches his shoulder and waits for her remark which comes very succinctly and quickly 'There is no chair here for me, there is no place in this room for me, I am only in the way.' The audience of patients waits tensely waiting for his response. I wait long enough to satisfy myself that he has received the meaning of her double. 'Well George, what do you think? Do you think you should say that to any one in this room? Do you want to say it to any one?' George takes a deep breath. Audrey is still in her place, close to him, touching his shoulder. 'I think I should say it to dad.' There is a pause. It seems to go on for a long time and momentarily I am confused, but I wait. George continues. 'But I suppose he should say it to me. I would in his place. Cuckoo in the bloody nest . . . that's what I am!'

Blatner's comment is confirmed in the naive psychodrama of a working-class patient who has never read Freud or the story of Oedipus either and yet spontaneously and quite unconsciously repeats the Oedipal myth in his dramatization. Blatner (1973) in his chapter 'Integration with other psychotherapeutic approaches' associated psychodramatic method with central psychodynamic concerns from various schools of theory. He wrote

> I consider the various theoretical systems of psychotherapy, and their practical methodologies as being essentially compatible with each other. Each approach relates to only a few facets of human experience, and a flexible application of several different methods may be required in the individualised treatment of each case. Moreover the synthesis of two methods often can result in significantly greater effectiveness than could be obtained from either method being used alone.

In the scene that I have described I mentioned my own confusion in George's silence. I had to silence myself, to restrain my anxious voice that wanted to speak for George. My countertransference was palpable. I did not trust George, dependent, inadequate George, to speak up for himself. Fortunately, I quelled the impulse and let George get on with the work himself. Sometimes new arrivals at the scene of psychodrama ask how the dynamics of countertransference and transference manifest themselves in the action of the drama? Well this seemed to me to be an obvious example. I brought it into the sharing at the closure of the group. I notice that Blatner appears not to deal with the issue of how far the director shares with the group at the closure. In this instance the material I offered to the group, in the sharing process, focused upon the anxiety the group felt when witnessing George's struggle to manage the furniture in setting up the scene. His inadequacy was felt to be compelling and seductive; I had experienced it in common with other group members and so I brought it back, tactfully, to their attention at the appropriate moment.

Scene 11

A lecture hall in Vienna. Sigmund Freud is giving his fifth lecture on psychoanalysis. The hall is full and there is an air of tense expectation. Let us imagine the following scene.

Freud faces a sceptical audience composed mostly of experienced doctors, some his critical rivals. He is dealing with the thorny issue of 'transference', that most provocative element in the doctor/patient relationship. He looks at the assembled audience and speaks: 'You may not suppose, moreover, that the phenomenon of transference is created by psycho-analytic influence. Transference arises in all human relationships just as it does between patient and physician.' There is an uneasy shuffling in the hall and a few semi-audible mutters of concern may be heard. Freud continues: 'It is everywhere the true vehicle of therapeutic influence; the less its presence is suspected, the more powerfully it operates.' Murmurs are now louder.

It is this last emphasis upon the unconscious and its place in the therapeutic relationship that excites most anxiety and attention. Freud pauses. He looks keenly at his audience before proceeding. He is in good form today, enjoying himself, speaking as usual, without notes.

At a later stage of this book I shall be considering the role of the director more closely and specifically but for now I wish merely to emphasize the place of the director as a member of the psychodrama group in which she receives and transmits both conscious and unconscious messages. In the more passive analytic group the reserved position of the leader makes it relatively easy for the trained therapist to monitor her own performance in the group and to keep under pretty firm control spontaneous impulses of speech and body movement. For the psychodrama director the problem is much more difficult as she performs her role with much more obvious speech and body movements, all of which will be interpreted by the group. Kellermann (1992) discusses the issues of transference in some depth. His article keeps very much to a theoretical position and, unfortunately, does not provide case study material to illustrate his views, but he does draw attention to Moreno's position where Moreno insists, quite rightly in my view, that: 'sometimes a patient is attracted by a therapist and another type of behaviour arises within the patient, as well as transference behaviour . . . another process in also active.'

He sees this as the patient discovering the 'real self' of the therapist. The term he uses to describe this process is *tele*. This seems to me inevitable.

The active psychodrama director cannot ultimately hide her 'real self'. By 'real self' I take it Moreno is referring to aspects of the director's personality that become absolutely apparent during the dramatic process. Just as the analytic group conductor has a therapy role to perform, which calls upon her to hide any spontaneous display of her own feelings and ideas so the psychodrama director has a role that allows her feelings and ideas to be channelled through the action of the protagonist and the audience in a much more obvious way. This does not mean that the director should simply manipulate the action; rather, the opposite is the therapeutic imperative. The dramatic play needs to be monitored all the time by the director to ensure that the spontaneity of the protagonist and group is not suppressed in favour of the desires of the director. When the director succeeds in doing this to the benefit of the protagonist then feelings of empathy and affection can easily follow and should be seen as appropriate. Similarly a piece of good work done against difficult odds can excite admiration and affection from the group and the director. I have certainly experienced this feeling myself and regarded it as a genuine response to a brave effort on the part of a group member, whether it be male or female.

Scene 12

The clinical psychology department of a large teaching, research mental hospital in St Petersburg, Russia. It is the time of Gorbachev. About 12 trainees are sitting in a large circle in the treatment room of the department. A young man is performing his psychodrama. He has flown down from Siberia to be present. By profession, although a psychologist, he is the director of a small experimental theatre company in a provincial town. At this point of the psychodrama he is in great distress. He has been married six months and he is working on the problem of the relationship with his wife.

Vladimir: 'She wants sex, nothing but sex, that is all she wants, nothing else. It's terrible. She does not love me. She just wants me to fuck her. That's all.'

Director: 'Speak to her Vladimir, speak to her directly, don't complain to me, speak to her, she is here with you.'

V: 'I can't! It's impossible! Only you seem to understand this situation. You, and the group.'

Alla (in role as his wife) tries to speak to him.

Alla: 'But Vladimir, my darling child, I do love you, please, its not just sex; let us make love. I love you so much.'

V (tears are now streaming down his face): 'You understand, Don, how much I struggle and suffer. Please!'

Director: 'Does she, do you think? Does your wife understand? Ask her Vladimir. Why don't you reverse role with her Vladimir?'

Vladimir absolutely refuses to do so. He is locked into a desperate inner conflict which he is defending as hard as he can and he is constantly looking to me to help, at the same time resisting my direction and the interventions of the group.

To categorize his behaviour as belonging exclusively to the realms of 'tele' or 'transference' is very difficult – the two are sometimes intertwined. But I am moved by his dilemma. I feel as if he has come on this long journey and he is looking to me for help that goes beyond merely my technical competence as a director. As a consequence when we meet the next day I ask the group if we can continue the work with Vladimir. At first they are somewhat surprised, but after a discussion, agree that this is how we will proceed. Vladimir looks grateful. I notice, too, that Alla, the woman playing his wife, looks pleased. In the work that then ensues he illustrates his dependent needs, his fear of failure in his masculinity, together with his terror of being taken over by women, reflecting his intrusive mother and weak, absent father.

Let me be brave and indicate some of the 'transference' brought to the director of the group that may be far from helpful. Yalom (1975) states: 'As long as a leader assumes responsibility of leadership, transference will occur. I have never seen a group without a rich and complex underpinning of transference. The problem is not of evocation but, on the contrary, resolution of transference.'

Like Yalom I think the therapy group, will, like a family, endow the leader with parental power and authority. The task, then, of the director is to resolve the transference so that members of the group are made aware of any distortions that may have occurred in their behaviour towards her. For example:

- Sometimes the director will experience excessive deference and excessive valuation of her skill and understanding. This disempowers the group and encourages dependency and helplessness. The members become deskilled.
- Rivalry may develop between members of the group for the favours of the director, real or imagined. Who, then, is the favourite member/son or daughter? The most rewarded or least rewarded performer in the dramas?
- The struggle for power. Who is in charge? Who lays down the rules and enforces them? Resulting confusion and hostility, deserved or otherwise, is aimed towards the director.
- Anxiety and accompanying fear of the director's attention. The therapy can be seen as persecutory and damaging.
- There are many more variations of these features of the relationship between director and group but most of them relate to these I have described.

In psychodrama transference resolution is not so much resolved by what the director says, in an interpretative way, but rather by the way she behaves towards the group. Not that the director is required to be mute in this matter.

Thus the director will tackle the distortions I have outlined by encouraging opposite attitudes and behaviour in the group. For example, dependency in the group is challenged by the director encouraging independence and originality in the group, manifested by individuals and by group attitudes. Similarly, favouritism is discouraged by the director being very even handed and encouraging towards all the individuals in the group whatever the level of their skills and performance. So the clumsiest performers get their chance and the clever entertaining actors have to wait their turn. On the issue of power, collective discussion of issues facing the group and decisions being reached by mutual agreement puts the power into the group and relieves the director of the burden of dictatorial control. Sometimes therapy that is challenging can appear to be persecutory. The best means of dealing with this situation is to bring it out into the group for healthy critical appraisal and discussion.

Finally, let us consider the countertransference feelings that may occur in a director. I demonstrated in my vignette concerning the patient 'George' how I faced countertransference feelings and dealt with them as best as I could. On the other hand my anxiety about torture and sadism, in another group, sprang not from countertransference but rather from issues belonging to me, not fully resolved. Sometimes the platitudes of psychotherapy sound as if all pathological issues can be resolved. This has not been my experience. These feelings I had, connected with sadistic persecution, were not intrinsically founded in my relationship with the patient concerned. As for 'undeserved love', as Freud sometimes called it, in respect of a client or patient in the group I have always found it relatively easy to identify such feelings and acknowledge to myself its presence with curiosity. When the director becomes self consciously aware of such a relationship emerging in the group, dealing with it becomes a matter of professional behaviour, making sure that the favoured one doesn't get special attention either in the group or outside of it. Countertransference, like transference, becomes damaging to the work of a psychodrama group when it is undetected and remains in the unconscious or preconscious, unacknowledged and hence unreasonably influential. The best resolution for a director is found in supervision, where it is available.

This chapter has been about psychodrama as group work where the individual, the protagonist, has a powerful presence, probably unique to the practice of psychodrama and as such attracts a value which can hardly be overstated. Within the group the psychodrama director has a very special place; she is the possessor of skills and therapeutic understanding but it should always be remembered that, as with all psychotherapists, she is there to serve the clients and should always work in the spirit of self-denial so that the group may benefit as a whole. My view is that if this advice is followed then nothing but good will come from it. As Professor Petruska Clarkson stated in a winter workshop flyer of December 1999: 'Research has shown that one of the most influential factors determining therapeutic outcome . . . is the quality of the relation between therapist and client; theoretical differences between schools are found to be relatively less important.'

I think Sue Jennings (1973) was right in associating therapy with emotional learning and in the next chapter this process will be approached and described.

Chapter 3

Learning in the psychodrama therapy group

'Wearing all that weight of learning lightly like a flower.'

Tennyson *In Memoriam*

In this chapter I want to address the issue of experiential learning, which is what every psychodrama trainee director does in the process of becoming a psychotherapist. I include different forms and levels of learning such as *emotional* learning, leading to insight and understanding, *cognitive* learning, which takes the learner into the literature and theories of psychotherapy and psychology, and *skills* learning where the trainee learns to exercise methods of working therapeutically. I shall look at the same phenomena as far as the psychodrama 'patient' or 'client' is concerned, but let us first address the path that leads to the role of director.

Here, at the beginning of this chapter, it is important to recognize the importance, in Britain, of the British Psychodrama Association (BPA), which has become, after years of struggle and development, the main agency for validating training in this country. Any aspiring psychodrama psychotherapist will eventually need to know about this body and register with one of its affiliated training organizations, in order to train and qualify as a therapist, duly recognized by the BPA and recommended by that body to the register of the United Kingdom Council for Psychotherapy (UKCP). The UKCP is, for the moment, the main registration body to which most aspiring psychotherapists turn for approval and recognition. As yet there is no statutory registration of psychotherapists in this country.

Some ten years ago the BPA was in its infancy and psychodrama was regarded by most mental health practitioners as a somewhat exotic and not altogether dependable way of practising psychotherapy. Today the situation is quite different and with the development of training has come the establishment of psychodrama as a mainstream therapy, with a growing presence as a therapy alongside the other psychotherapies practised in the National Health Service, or privately. At the end of the book I have given the contact address for the BPA, which is a good starting place for those interested in going into formal training, or those who wish at this stage to join and become part of the 'scene' as it were, where they can become acquainted with psychodramatist therapists and trainers.

Another introductory approach to becoming a psychodramatist, which probably comes before formal training, is to go to a few workshops and then open up the subject through reading, the cognitive part of the self. This book will help in that respect and I have already mentioned the excellent work by Anthony Williams (1989) and especially Kellermann (1992), to which I shall be referring throughout this book. There also exists a basic introduction by David Brazier (1994) and there is *What is Psychodrama?* by Derek Gale (1995) – very much a beginner's book. Perhaps the weightiest of these British introductory texts is *Psychodrama: Inspiration and Technique* edited by Paul Holmes and Marcia Karp (1991). Marcia Karp is the founder of the most important training organization in this country and she is, at the time of writing, the Honorary President of the BPA. Her influence is felt and disseminated throughout the world of psychodrama by the many psychodramatists that have trained with her and her partner Ken Sprague, a sociodramatist. At the back of this book the reader will find a fuller bibliography and the names and addresses of the present training bodies and where and how to contact them. At this point I wish to turn to the more subjective elements of training to become a psychodramatist.

In Chapter 2 I already referred, in passing, to the training of the psychodrama director. Readers will have picked up the view that I am not too keen on short-lived, ephemeral experiences in the 'training group'. In contrast to the training of group and individual psychoanalytic psychotherapists and, of course, psychoanalysts, the training of psychodramatists in England has tended towards short, intensive experiences centred upon weekend training, supplemented by occasional workshops. I would stress that this is not always so and a number of training courses now facilitate sustained continuous training courses. But many therapists have found their way towards psychodrama that way. My own experience was rather of that character. Following sustained group therapy where I had been in the same group as a 'patient' for some two years and then for another year, where the membership was stable and continuous, meeting on a weekly basis and where no one left the group in the lifetime of the group, I was introduced to a much less stable formation: a psychodrama training group coming into being. At first the group was rather 'wobbly' – we were never sure who would be present. I found this worrying. Others seemed not to be especially concerned. Entry to the group was entirely voluntary and without any selection. I think this is actually quite a good way of getting a group together. I am sceptical of advance selection, exclusion and inclusion. We were essentially a group of 'patients' coming together with a highly skilled psychodramatist and co-therapist, a highly talented man and woman respectively, to learn and to experience the therapy of psychodrama. The meetings of the group were rather infrequent but very intensive. We met on a weekend basis, some of us staying in hotels for at least a couple of nights. The group then met for all the time available, allowing for meal breaks but continuing, sometimes from ten in the morning until about seven or eight at night – a lot of hours. If meeting at weekends is the only way that such a group may be organized then I think this use of time, although somewhat exhausting for directors and members of the group alike, is preferable to shorter, less intense sessions. And so, reader, if you are looking for initial training, be prepared! This may be your experience. You may well have to put up with the unavoidable and avoidable absence of group members and a somewhat shifting population of group membership, experiencing the distortions that then may arise. However, over the course of time, my training group did finally become most cohesive and regular in its attendance, which I found to be a comfort.

Scene 13

Ten trainees in a training group gather for a weekend of training in a residential set up. Marjorie has failed to turn up again. We are all annoyed, except perhaps the director. 'She is broke', he kindly explains. 'She has no money and can't pay. We say come anyway, but she will not. There is not a thing we can do about it.' Several of the group look distinctly annoyed. I find jealousy welling up inside of me. The director obviously thinks Marjorie is the 'bees knees'. Would he allow me to come without paying? Why doesn't he get rid of her? Why doesn't he make it a condition of group membership that she comes regularly? I think I know why. He is really fed up that she hasn't come because he thinks she is probably the most talented person in the group. And she is good at directing; so imaginative, quick to respond and generally getting to the heart of the matter with flair and talent. So he loves her best and will put up with her inconstancy. So be it. Several other members of the group and I are not pleased. But nothing is said.

Nothing is said or explored because the director, in this instance, doesn't open up any exploration of the feelings of the group about Marjorie and her place in our small world of training. But, whether the director acknowledges it or not, the situation for the group was as I have described it. The trainees in this instance may simply gossip about it outside the framework of the training sessions. Trainee psychodramatists in such a setting may well experience this or similar discontent and discomfort. If time and attention is given to their feelings then time has to be found within the structure of the therapy group to process the material. Much rests upon the orientation and skill of the director. Obviously, there is an opportunity for individual and group learning in such an experience as described but the moment has to be right and it is impossible to prescribe in advance how and when this emotional learning should be addressed.

Compared with a group analytic group a psychodrama group cannot be so tightly time bound. The analytic group will finish on the hour precisely and many a member, at first experiencing this, is shocked by the sometimes abrupt manner such a group will close a session, before meeting again. But the psychodrama group has to work through a structure of coming together, finding a protagonist and a theme, finding a dramatization, performing it, and then resolving some of the issues in a group sharing and closure. A lot has to be done. If issues of transference are to be dealt with then time for that has to be found as well. So we are talking about two or three hours of work or even longer. Moreno (1923) describes the complexity of the psychodrama performance:

> The dramas in which we are interested are not those which mature in the minds of artists but long before they reach them as they spring up in everyday life, in the minds of simple people. We deal with the drama at a level where the neat separation of the aesthetic from the therapeutic is meaningless. The actors are not any people, but our people, our fathers and mothers, our brothers and sisters, friends and neighbours . . . catharsis moves from spectator to the actor and from the actor back to the spectator.

This is a highly subtle and subjective experience and time has to be made for its process. So although we may have a notion of the ending and closure of the psychodrama group it has to be approached with these constraints in mind. There can be no abrupt ending with the director simply calling halt and leaving. Notice how Moreno is foreshadowing what Brecht speaks about when he talks about the drama of the streets, referred to in Chapter 1.

Other training may be available as a less fragmented and continuous learning experience and I have run training groups for as long as a year at a time, on a week-by-week basis, which I believe to be the preferred method. In such a setting time can be found for considering transference issues. Sometimes a direct approach is required but, more often, the distortions that may be attributed to transference may be resolved in action. As the weeks go by with a steady and consistent attendance there can be a carry-over of experience, a historical dialogue develops where members of the group may reflect backwards to earlier material without too much difficulty. This is one of the advantages of the continuing group. Quite obviously, skills learning is enhanced too, as trainees have more opportunities to practice and gain confidence as protagonists, alter egos and directors. The whole host of therapy roles is rehearsed again and again.

Transference, in particular, may be addressed and resolved, within such a timeframe, as much through *group action*, as through *dialogue* with the director. As well as the transference relationship it should be remembered that another type of relationship with the director is possible. Moreno (1959) recognized this when he writes about *tele*, although the term is often used in a muddled and inconsistent manner. He described it as 'a mutual exchange of empathy and appreciation', a kind of 'therapeutic love'. Sometimes this is spoken of by psychotherapists as the 'therapeutic alliance', which develops between therapist and client and is seen as non pathological and not embedded in 'transference'. Rogers (1969) speaks of the: 'warm, subjective human meeting between two people'. It seems to me that such a situation is likely to develop when the group is not transient and has time to grow and to establish confidence in itself and the director.

Scene 14

St Petersburg in the former Soviet Union. A training group in Psychodrama has been convened in a major hospital for the treatment of mental disorders. This is my third year in St Petersburg working with a group of Russian doctors and psychologists, some of whom have attended all the sessions up to now.

I am the trainer. Disaster faces us on day one when it becomes apparent that my trusted collaborator and translator has abandoned the course without notice. He has abandoned the group and me. The group is very angry. I decide to ask the group to discuss the issue, without me being present, and then we will join together to see what we can achieve in his new and critical situation. I too am dismayed and angry. This group was planned to meet daily for about six weeks and I am established in a flat in the city with my wife in support as my 'minder'. When I tell my wife, she takes a softer line concerning my 'betrayal.' As it turns out my collaborator, who has worked with me for some years, has been invited at the last moment to go to Paris to a conference, all expenses paid, at the invitation of UNESCO. Such seduction he cannot resist! He has never before in his life had an opportunity to visit Paris.

The Russians in the group are not accustomed to the responsibility of facing up to making a decision without the 'leader' guiding them to a conclusion that suits her. The next day we meet again. They have a spokesman – Igor, a psychiatrist of some standing.

He announces: 'Natasha, who speaks virtually perfect English and is an experienced clinical psychologist will translate and work with you.'

I listen and say: 'She will be paid.'

Spoken as statement rather than a question. We go on to discuss this 'fly in the ointment' that I have introduced and eventually resolve it in her favour. She smiles and quickly and efficiently translates the entire debate to me as it takes place. I note that, although she had gained in status and money by taking on this role as my translator and co-therapist, she has lost the position of 'patient' and this must be addressed in due course. Some other compensation will have to be found.

This sustained group, meeting on a regular basis, with some degree of frequency, has many advantages and not least among them is the fact that illusions and fantasies about other group members and their apparent capabilities and power are soon exposed for what they are, the anxieties we all share concerning our own inadequacies. Group morale is built and trust is evidenced and so the possibilities of the psychodrama group are extended and group interaction becomes less competitive and more cooperative. Solutions are found for what appear at first to be intractable problems. The learning, which is primarily emotional, is powerful.

Scene 15

A training group for would-be psychodramatists in the mid 1980s. The setting is a mental hospital in the north of England. The group is sitting in a comfortable room, somewhat overheated, lounging in deep armchairs.

Joan has settled down into her armchair and has apparently suddenly dropped off to sleep. She does this from time to time. The group has been in existence for some two years.

Jane: *'Wakey, wakey Joan'. Come on you are not going off to sleep now. We know you are tired. We all are, so come on wake up.*

Joan: *'Oh come off it, leave me alone, I am exhausted. Two hours of psychodrama are knackering and it took me two hours to drive here.'*

Jim: *'No way Joan, come on. We are all in the same boat. Come on this is our sharing time and we don't want to hear your snores. They are no substitute for what you need to say to us.'*

The rest of the group murmur and join in with muffled 'hear hears'.

Dave: 'I've had enough of this. Let's get on with it. Joan you are showing off! Look, she's wide awake now, not that she was ever asleep.'

This is simply a recording of the kind of risky interchange that becomes possible in a group that feels safe and bonded together. No one sulks or loses temper. People are open and frank with each other and are prepared to take reasonable risks in their relationships to their mutual benefit. The lesson is that the psychodrama has not ended with the performance – on the contrary the performance lingers in the interchange that Moreno describes and is processed in the relationships of the members of the group. In this instance everyone knows that Joan will, given half a chance, simply go off into a gentle non-intrusive, non-participative doze when the topic grows threatening. But this ambivalence will give way to the challenge where her defensiveness is tackled by trusted members of the group. Notice that the director had no need to intervene in this 'little drama'. She could let the group get on with it knowing that they could handle it with ease. The group has learned how to handle itself.

Many years ago, as a young student, I read J.A.C. Brown (1950) and saw described, for the first time, the developing stages of the group that meets together on a regular basis. I remember it to this day. Brown spoke of the group 'forming, storming, norming and performing', which seems very appropriate to what can commonly be observed in the learning and developing psychodrama group.

Perhaps at this point it is worth stating in clear terms what divides the experience of the trainee from that of the 'patient' or 'client' in the psychodrama group. It starts with the basic conscious motivation of each category. No matter how mixed the motives, bearing in mind that sometimes we enter training to mask our need for therapy, which for a number of reasons we may be ashamed to acknowledge, the trainee has made a decision to become a psychodramatist. The way is clear. A condition is that she joins a psychodrama group in which to experience being a 'client' and at the same time learn about the content and method of the psychodrama group, which is very special and particular and can only be properly learned from practical experience.

So from the very beginning there is a complex presence of therapy and training, which incorporates some formal cognitive and skills as well as emotional learning. The weight of each presence will be felt in varying degrees according to the process and character of the group. The trainee may move from at one moment being the 'patient' who has worked dramatically as the protagonist, through some very intense and personal material to, on another occasion, being required to direct a psychodrama of one of her companions in the group. When this occurs then virtually all levels of learning are activated in the service of the protagonist. The latter is essential if the trainee is going to acquire directorial skills at the level to make her a caring, competent and skilful psychodramatist.

At the same time this shift from patient to director is viewed by the trainer/director and judged professionally, as to whether the skill of the aspiring director is good enough to serve the end of the protagonist. This requirement to judge must have an impact upon the relationship between trainee and director. It is perfectly proper that such a critical, evaluating relationship should exist. But, of course, this places the trainee in a very different position from that of a person who is in the psychodrama group entirely for personal therapeutic reasons. This juxtaposition of role is inevitable and traditional. The trainee director is going to need to demonstrate not only the technical skills of direction but the deeper, subtler use of psychological understanding and interpretation. Much is required of her. Thus the 'training group' is very different from the 'therapy group', although both will share common elements, and it is possible for therapeutic experience to exist in both. It is a matter of balance and role. It is very necessary to be clear both in the training situation and in the therapy group.

In respect of other training therapies it is very different. For example, when in an analytic training group I was always the 'patient' and I was never required to be the analyst in that group. My clinical experience as the group analyst took place in an entirely different setting, where I worked as a co-therapist. In individual psychoanalytic training the training therapist is in a much more, but not entirely, 'pure' position than the psychodrama director conducting a training group. The training therapist, like the psychodrama trainer, will inevitably be seen as a model by the trainee. The extent and significance of this will vary a great deal from one trainee to another.

Unfortunately, at the present time, the opportunities are very limited for persons wanting to enter a therapeutic psychodrama group. There are very few private groups and most groups are provided in psychotherapy centres within the National Health Service or the private institutions offering psychotherapy as a treatment. I think that the best approach to finding a private group would be to use the directory of the United Kingdom Council for Psychotherapy where all trained and fully competent psychodamatists are registered. Most psychodramatists know of each other and can recommend sources of group therapy when they are unable, personally, to provide such a service for clients.

In contrast to the experience of the trainee psychodramatist, the client in a therapeutic group will not have to encounter the professional judgement of the psychodramatist in the training role. In that respect both the 'tele' aspects of the relationship and the 'transference' aspects are clearer and less ambiguous, to the benefit of the individual and the group as a whole. The client in a psychodrama therapy group will certainly 'learn' about the techniques of the psychodrama group process. Indeed it is an imperative, so that all the other members of the group may gain benefit. The therapy is group therapy. The importance of the therapeutic learning lies at a profound, emotional and cognitive level. There is often a shift in the position of a client in the process of the group, a corrective emotional experience as it is sometimes called, that leads to learning that in turn leads to a new attitude and the opportunity for new behaviour. This behaviour can often be observed by members of the group in the group and commented upon by the client in terms of relationships 'outside' the group. This 'learning' is never assessed in the terms that the trainee will experience because it is essentially restricted to the life of the group and its members as individuals. The only other interested party is the therapist. But the therapist is not required to use the information for anything other than therapeutic purposes.

Of course there are not always good outcomes or creative processes in psychodrama. Sometimes there is a cathartic shift of feeling that becomes a corrective emotional experience for the protagonist, but sometimes the process fails. Two examples illustrate this point.

Scene 16

A clinical psychodrama group meeting weekly in a therapy centre. They meet in the evening in a large room. Ill lit and under ventilated, it smells from the use it has had all day. Cigarette ends flow out of ashtrays. Used tissues are strewn around the floor. A number of harsh strip lights cast a cold worn out look upon somewhat shabby furniture. The group is assembling, pushing armchairs together to form a circle. The director has not yet arrived.

Mary, who is never late, sits alone in the circle. A few other members stand around, apparently a little reluctant to sit down with Mary. One of them, John, in defiance of the notice on the wall is 'finishing off a fag'.

The director enters. The group sits down. A seat remains empty beside Mary.

Twenty minutes later and as yet no one has asked to become the protagonist for the evening.

John: 'I don't know what we are waiting for. Everyone here except Mary has done a psychodrama.'

There is a silence. Mary sighs.

Jennifer: 'She will when she is ready.'

Harry: 'When will that be?'

John (whispers, barely audibly): 'God knows!'

Mary looks around the group but there is little eye contact from the rest of the group.

Mary: 'I have been thinking about it. But I honestly can't think of a real issue. You know something really important.'

The director: 'Perhaps I can help. Shall we have a talk, Mary?'

Mary nods but says nothing. The director asks her if he may sit in the empty seat beside her. She nods but does not speak. The director leaves his chair and crosses the room. He pauses beside Mary, who looks up at him, and then sits down.
As he does so the co-therapist walks across the room and stands behind Mary's chair and touches her shoulder firmly but lightly.

Co-therapist: 'I'm doubling for you Mary.'

There is a pause and a silence. Mary gives the briefest of nods. Her eyes look at the floor. The co-therapist continues speaking for Mary.

Co-therapist: 'I'm feeling really scared now. It's going to happen. She is sitting beside me, which means that I'm really in for it. Oh my god!'

At this point Mary's shoulders begin to shake. Her eyes begin to fill with tears and small sobs begin to escape from her body. There is long silence.

Jennifer: 'Are you OK, Mary? Shall we stop? Are you OK, are you?'

Mary: 'Yes, yes, of course I'M OK. It's just that I have been so silly. I couldn't speak before. I don't know if I can now.'

She continues to sob quietly, then with a big effort she begins to stand up.

The director: 'Are you sure you want to go on? You don't have to. You know it's your decision.'

Mary looks at the director and gives a wan smile and nods. Now she moves to the middle of the circle and pulling out a tissue sneezes, wipes her eyes and coughs. 'OK,' she says. 'Where shall I start?'

Director: 'Anywhere you like. Let's take a little walk and then you can talk to me, yeah you can talk to all of us.'

He is standing beside Mary now and briefly touches her elbow; they start to walk around the circumference of the group.

So the psychodrama begins with every promise of a therapeutic encounter and outcome, but it is not always so and the next scene taken from a similar group in a similar setting gives another picture of life in a psychodrama group.

Scene 17

A psychodrama group that has only been in existence for a few weeks. The clients are mostly very disturbed individuals, most of them with a long psychiatric history. The group is balanced between five men and five women. They are in early middle age and their social class is very mixed ranging from middle-class professional to working-class, unskilled. The group is sitting quietly, waiting for the director/psychotherapist and co-therapist to arrive. There is very little talk, just two of the women are whispering to each other. A smart woman, Janet, in her mid-forties, dressed in a dark fashionable suit, sits, her body turned away from the group, looking out of the window, which is dirty, begrimed and only allowing the briefest glint of sunshine into the room. She is distancing herself in a blatant disassociative manner. The whispering women glance at her from time to time. Perhaps they envy her clothes, leather handbag and boots. Janet is reading a paperback book, probably a 'good' novel.

The director arrives with his co-therapist; they both notice Janet's behaviour. They join the group and look around. Janet continues to read ignoring the director and the group.

Director: 'Good morning everyone.'

There is a quiet response, mere whispering of greeting from members of the group. Janet continues to read her book. Her concentration is exclusively with the text. She makes no acknowledgement of the director or the implication of his presence. The director looks around, notes that everyone is present and that Janet is still reading her book. He glances at the co-therapist who pauses, takes a breath and speaks: 'Janet we are here to start the psychodrama group.' Silence. Janet continues to read.

Here we have a group that is facing a serious neurotic problem in one of its members that is not being directly addressed but is being 'enacted' by the member concerned, Janet. Until the denial and defence is addressed and resolved the group cannot move into any kind of creative action. The irony is that this is just the sort of problem that could be worked upon with productive results in psychodrama if the protagonist will enter the group with a determination to address the issues hidden behind the resistance. In this case, however, Janet stays stubbornly entrenched in her refusal to work creatively against the neurosis that entraps her. This situation remained as it is described until the director decided to ask the group as a whole to confront the dilemma of Janet's behaviour, which they did, albeit with some hesitation and reluctance. They know from their learning experience in the group that their intervention is critical and essential. Janet used the most simplistic and unrealistic defence trying to insist that the group 'get on without me, I don't mind, I'm quite happy to go on reading my book.'

Many trainees in psychodrama never encounter such situations in their experience of training, and when they do in a clinical situation they are 'stumped'. What are they to do? My view is quite straightforward. The psychodrama group is a therapy group first and foremost and the members of the group need to be active in dealing with any attack upon the life of the group. This is a theoretical position that the director has to have learned in her training. How she will tackle it will vary from one director to another and with the different dynamics of the group, but tackle it she must.

A good account of a clinical psychodrama group struggling with the problem of a member's resistance and anxiety at the prospect of working with the group is contained in Widlake (1997) where psychodramatist Bernard Widlake describes an experience with a patient he calls Barbara, a young adult recovering from an eating disorder. Barbara evidences a marked ambivalence, which she shows to the group in the form of 'wanting and not wanting' to work psychodramatically, whilst at the same time participating in group life with a sense of commitment in various warm-up exercises and playing roles in other people's dramas. Bernard

Widlake does not identify the behaviour as 'resistance': rather he talks about her ambivalence and nervousness.

The term 'resistance' is an early Freudian concept. Freud noticed that although his clients came to him for assistance, they were frequently afraid of revealing 'too much' concerning their personal traumas and difficulties in relationships. They were sometimes ashamed of their experience or felt guilty concerning thoughts and feelings they had harboured towards others, or even dismayed at their actual behaviour, which they saw as deceiving and lacking in genuineness. Could they trust Freud? Of course Freud was working entirely individually with these patients and he soon realized that he had to address these defensive postures himself if the patient was going to make any progress.

In the psychodrama group run by Bernard Widlake he had the immense advantage of working with the group and the group process engendering trust, risk taking and openness. His client by the fifth session of the group is able to move into the role of protagonist. After the sixth session she leaves. I will have more to say about this and the issue of time in psychodrama at a later point in this book.

Although the process of resolution in the group is very different from the position in individual psychoanalytic psychotherapy, the issue of defence and resolution remains the same. Bernard worked patiently and sensitively with her to help her overcome her 'resistance' with some success. In her final session the young woman in the case study actually apologized to the group for her earlier behaviour with them. The members are recorded here as saying the apology was not necessary, but my view is that therapeutically speaking the apology could have been seen as important evidence of her emotional learning and consequent shift of attitude. Barbara herself kept a session-by-session written account of this experience in a psychodrama group and I end this chapter with some quotations from her 'diary'.

> [Interview with Bernard before joining the group:] what do I know about this man . . . how much shall I let him know . . . must be careful he doesn't see through me first . . . he's onto something and I'm on to something . . .
>
> [About the members of the group:] Don't get too close. Can't participate with others. Don't they understand. Tried to convince others that they were weak and gullible for being brainwashed and manipulated (by Bernard). But really just sick with myself for being so resistant . . .

In the end positive transference and good 'tele' won out and Barbara learned how to confront and deal with her resistances; moving into therapeutic action. It should be noticed that she employed her 'cognitive' aspect, her language skill, in the form of a written diary of events, to support her exploration of the therapeutic struggle. Closing this chapter on this hopeful note the realist in me directs the reader to accept that all therapies have their limitations. This view will be addressed in the next chapter.

CHAPTER 4

What can and cannot be achieved

Hope springs eternal

In this chapter I shall be concerned with what can reasonably be achieved through the practice of psychodrama and its techniques. I shall also consider limitations in relation to other forms of psychotherapy, especially individual psychotherapy or counselling.

For the most part I am thinking of psychodrama being a 'group' activity whereas I know, at another level, it is quite capable of being used in an individual encounter and is sometimes used that way by practitioners who find themselves without a group with which to work. Or sometimes it may be used this way by preference.

Scene 18

The setting is my therapy room in a Georgian town house some 200 years old. It is late afternoon; the light is quietly leaving the sky. The room is warm and comfortable. Emily is sitting in front of me ruminating on the past. She is really in a kind of trance, a hypnotic state. I am merely the listener to what is essentially an internal dialogue. She is remembering an orchard in which she used to play. She remembers her father, a pleasant, secure presence in her life as a child. He too is in the orchard quietly pruning some small saplings. Her voice is low and comforting. I can easily hear her in my silence, which I maintain. Suddenly there is a change of tone, a change of sound, of voice. The warm, well-modulated voice has gone and has been replaced with a screech:

'Come in Emily, come in this instant! What on earth do you think you are doing? Just look at your dress! It's filthy! Ruined! I don't know what your father can be thinking of. Come in, NOW, straight away.' The mother is almost beside herself with jealous anger.

Notice how close this memory is to the example of the tearful man and his mother that I gave earlier in the book. This is an example of an involuntary psychodramatic moment. I did not call it forth or contrive its presence; it came quite spontaneously from the memory of my client, who had heard that voice inside herself for many years, a silent, internal forceful voice of reprimand, disapproval and judgement. I simply let it happen. My response was, after a suitable pause, merely to say: 'your mother'. Emily nodded and the session proceeded.

Moreno spoke about the possibility of conducting psychodrama within individual pychotherapy. John Casson (1997) quotes a 'tape' of Moreno describing the possibility of working *à deux* in contrast to the limitations of group psychotherapy, which can logically only be done in a group. But for most of us this is the exception rather than the rule. For the most part psychodrama is conducted in groups, either especially formed for the purpose or those groups that may occur organically within some sort of institutional framework, which are them brought into a psychodramatic context for a specific purpose. The obvious example would be a staff group which uses the psychodramatic approach to illustrate its social and psychological condition as a group with the purpose of, perhaps, bringing about change. I conducted such a group some years ago within a clinical psychology service.

As psychodrama psychotherapists we work for most of the time assuming that we are doing some good and avoiding the bad. We are attached to the benign and think we are working towards good outcomes for our clients. I think most of us take this for granted and rarely think otherwise about our work. We are also informed by ethical guidelines outlined by the BPA. However – and this is an important reservation – the truth is most of us do not bother to do any research to demonstrate that our beliefs are true. Indeed we appear to be indifferent to the discipline of research and unwilling to submit ourselves to the demands of research discipline and culture whether it be of the positivist scientific kind or the more creative participative sort. There is little in the way of research to demonstrate the implicit claims of our therapy. What evidence there is comes primarily from the United States, which is a country only deceptively like Britain, especially in its language. Roberta Kane (1992) writes with concern and critically of the manner that is adopted towards research in the world of psychodrama. Little attempt to use research methods is apparent and we rely upon the reporting of clinical experiences in a descriptive manner, rather than using an analytical research-based method in appraising the quality of our work. There is also an apparent indifference or unawareness existing towards the harm that unskilful psychodramatists may do their unwitting clients through inadequate or inappropriate interventions in what is generally recognized to be a very powerful therapeutic way of working with clients. There is little in the way of literature on the subject and the topic remains only occasionally addressed in professional journals or conferences. Blatner (1973) echoes the same concern and speaks of the absence of 'properly controlled outcome studies' in psychodrama.

Paul Wilkins (1997) writes about 'psychodrama and research' from a Rogerian background of training and affiliation. He starts by baldly stating that 'few studies demonstrates its [psychodrama's] usefulness or value' and quotes only some 30 research publications. This is amazing when it is realized that psychodrama, as a therapeutic tool, has been in active use now for over half a century. It confirms my belief that, as a profession, we are very reluctant to test ourselves in any empirical manner. Wilkins then goes on to suggest that we find ways of using psychodrama as a research tool. I think his idea is to try to use the creative elements in the psychodramatist towards successful research. He sees the benefits of such activity as being:

- helping us to gain wider perspectives and from this experience, learning and sharing that learning with others;
- becoming accountable for the usefulness and effectiveness of our therapy and as a protection of our profession from the vagaries of the abusive therapist;
- developing new ideas and approaches, which means opening ourselves up to the influence of other psychotherapeutic practice. This is a particular issue for all psychotherapists who appear, as a profession, to be very guarded and protective of the 'specialness' of their own particular approaches to therapy;
- the application of psychodrama to a variety of client groups, showing that we have a persuasive and effective way of working towards the benefit of disparate client groups;
- advancing and developing our professional development as individuals and as a profession.

With regard to this last suggestion, the UKCP is showing a good deal of interest in finding ways of defining continuing professional development with a view to introducing it into the professional structure of the practising professional psychotherapist. This is all very laudable but essentially untested in practice. And it may turn out to be impractical.

For the moment I am not going to pursue the issue of research any further except to note, in my own research of the literature, its sparcity, especially in the British context. Rather I would like to set out some obvious particulars that relate to the question 'what can and cannot be achieved through psychodrama?'

Given a psychodrama group and the presence of the protagonist then I believe that the following benefits may be attributed to the process of the therapy.

Psychodrama as a diagnostic tool

Psychodrama is an excellent diagnostic tool and a brilliant way of obtaining a case 'history'. The psychodramatic interview, with its mixture of conversation and dramatic expositions, quickly opens up key issues in the protagonist's life. Drama, by its very nature, is a means of telling a story and the protagonist soon finds she can tell her story fluently and vividly through the medium of the psychodramatic method.

The immediacy of psychodrama

The immediacy of psychodrama is one of its first virtues. Moving quickly into action expedites the therapeutic encounter.

Scene 19

A university seminar room. The client group consists entirely of trainee psychotherapists following a higher degree route towards practice. The director has come to offer insight into psychodrama. He has said he isn't going to conduct a psychodrama but rather illustrate its tools and approaches in a practical manner that the group can work with and explore. A quiet woman is following his introduction with great interest. He begins to talk about warming up character and suggests someone from the group could simply come into the middle of the circle, choose someone from the group to stand for a significant figure in their life, and then warm up the figure through the technique of 'doubling' – speaking as if for the person. He has already noted the interest of the woman in the group who gives the appearance of an attractive and 'open' figure, so he is not surprised when she volunteers and steps forward. She chooses another woman from the group, Joan.

She is clearly older than Sarah. She begins: 'This is my mother.'

The director intervenes: 'Hang on a moment Sarah. Speak as if you were your mother.'

Sara looks puzzled.

The director prompts her: 'Simply touch Jane lightly on the shoulder and start by saying "My name is, what ever it is. I am Sarah's mother", and so on.'

He pauses and looks enquiringly at Sara to see if she understands him.

Sara : 'Oh I see, OK. Here we go!'

And so Sarah starts the warm up. She speaks as if she were her mother. For a while. The information is all factual. Her mother is called Joan. Joan has three children, one boy and two girls. There is an absence of feeling. The director lets this carry on for some while and then intervenes again.

The director suddenly says quite firmly: 'And how do you feel about that? What are your feelings? We are not hearing much about your feelings. About your family Joan!' (Of course the resistance is in Sarah.)

In role, the tone and colour of the warm up changes quickly, Sarah speaks of mother's feelings towards the children in the family and the tensions concerning her husband. Sarah's eyes are now beginning to fill up with tears but she manages to keep the monologue going. Gradually she unfolds the character of her mother. Her mother's very strong feelings about the children especially about her, Sarah. The co-therapist alter ego stands close to her making the occasional intervention, supporting and assisting Sara in the process. The director brings the warm up gently to a close. He reminds the group that he has no intention of conducting the emerging psychodrama any further. For the moment he regards the works as being concluded. But it will almost certainly come back into frame again in the future. The group are surprised and appreciative of the speed and immediacy of the method and say so in the debriefing and sharing that concludes the session.

It might be thought that the presence of the figure playing 'mother' in the chair was redundant. But in reality her presence brought the palpable quality of the actual mother to the scene. In a developing psychodrama she (in role) might well have asked the protagonist questions about herself and facilitated more feeling material from Sarah. Her physical presence in the scene was powerful and the protagonist, being touched by the auxiliary, was activated emotionally and responded to the feelings inside herself.

How the protagonist and director cooperatively, working together, make use of the immediacy of this psychodramatic process, is what matters and is finally definitive of the value of the therapy; but nevertheless as a method it is quite remarkable in its ability to engage the client with such immediacy and emotional energy in the exploration of life issues.

The descriptive nature of psychodrama

Psychodrama is essentially descriptive. By this I mean that it has the character of good imaginative storytelling. The protagonist usually responds to a series of cues, coming either from her self, *inner arising*, or from *without*, that is from an *auxiliary* figure, the group or the director. For example, the *warming up* of a character for the benefit of an alter ego is essentially descriptive and usually, with help the protagonist, can offer a vivid physical, emotional and social description of a mother, father, sibling, partner or friend in a very short time. Similarly, simply laying out a family room, with its furniture and accessories and placing family members in the scene reveals much about family dynamics before a word is spoken.

Psychodrama and the expression of feeling

Many clients, coming to a therapist for help, wish to find an arena where feelings can be safely expressed, whatever they are. Psychodrama, by its very nature, encourages the protagonist client to discover and express feelings, not only as a safe release of tension, but as part of the therapeutic process of 'catharsis', 'working through' and 'resolution'. The manner in which this will be achieved will vary from one director to another and rarely are all three states experienced in the same session.

Action

Psychodrama allows and encourages action. Sometimes the action is tangible, shown in the context of feelings towards another significant person, or sometimes it is symbolic, displaced onto furniture or properties. For example, the tearing up of a love letter, the careful preparation of a room, obsessive attention to laying a table. Very few psychotherapies allow the client to 'act' or 'show' through action the quality of a relationship or the process of a significant event. Indeed 'action' in therapy is sometimes experienced by therapists as pathological, even threatening. Foulkes (1975) talks about 'suspended action' as a positive quality of abstinence. Unfortunately, I noticed in my work in a mental hospital where I worked, that 'acting out' by the patient, that is when the patient actually 'behaved distressed', the reaction from clinical staff was judgemental and condemning. The term had become a term of abuse. This is particularly unfortunate when it is remembered that psychotherapy has, perhaps as its first duty, to try to understand behaviour before any thought occurs of judgement or interpretation is attempted.

Scene 20

The therapist's consulting room. He is psychoanalytic in orientation. It is early morning. The therapist notices the suppressed state of his client as the client enters the room. He sits down. There is a dull silence. The client avoids eye contact. His eyes are fixed staring towards the wall. Silence. The therapist is wondering how to interpret or manage this unfolding situation. More silence. It is becoming hard for both the therapist and client to maintain the silence much longer.

The client speaks: 'I feel so fucking angry. I would like to smash your head in. Really smash it. It's OK for you sitting there. Yeah. I know it's not you, but I feel so angry, I just want to punch someone, so it may as well be you.'

The client raises both his fists and starts a violent shadow boxing, he breathes quickly and noisily as he does it. The therapist sits, quiet, apparently composed but in reality he is shaken by this demonstration. The shadow boxing gets closer and closer and the therapist is beginning to wonder if it will get out of control and the blows will fall upon him. The whole scene is unfamiliar to him, nothing like this has happened before and he fears for his safety. Suddenly the client stops. He looks a bit bewildered. 'Sorry about that.'

In contrast the psychodramatic method offers a safe framework for powerful action. Any skilled psychodramatist could have put the client, in this example, into a safe but emotionally freeing situation. Sometimes the action is symbolic. For example, the client can find objects to represent a person or an institution or a state of feeling and vent feelings toward it.

Scene 21

The conference room of a large Soviet teaching and research mental hospital. I am conducting a psychodramatic staff session in which the clinical staff work towards a better understanding of their relative relationships with each other both individually and as a group. I notice that none of the nursing staff are present and, indeed, when asked to attend they refused to do so. I ask any one in the group to choose any object in the room to represent the leadership of the hospital. A psychiatrist walks towards the end of the room where on a rather high fireplace ledge is a somewhat musty bronze figure of Lenin. He picks it up and carries it into the centre of the group and places it on the floor. There is a palpable silence in the group. I say 'Well, what now?'

A young woman clinical psychologist gets up, picks up the statue and takes it to the door and faces it outwards, towards the corridor outside. Another woman, older and grey, takes off her headscarf walks across and covers the statue with it. No one speaks. There is a pause. It is as if we are waiting for something significant to happen. The oldest psychiatrist, in his late sixties, lumbers to his feet, walks across to the bronze figure takes off the scarf, opens the door takes it outside, places it on the floor near the wall, returns to the room, closes the door, walks steadily to his chair and speaks: 'Well, perhaps now we can get started . . .' (he pauses ironically) . . . 'comrades'.

As I write this I recall it was only weeks before this incident that Gorbachev was arrested at his Black Sea dacha and prevented from talking to the people and Yeltsin stood on a tank outside the parliament building and rallied resistance to a Stalinist coup. So the issue of leadership, command and control was a hot one for everyone in that room, at that hospital. It was evident that, although pressed to attend the workshop by the clinical director of their department, the nurses felt too insecure to take any risks in a public situation and stayed away.

Psychodrama encourages resolution

Because the drama unfolds, often historically, there is a tendency to work toward a 'finale' where the protagonist may make a closing statement which acknowledges the work done, the insight gained and perhaps some affirmation concerning the future. This is not always so, of course – there is no rule that insists such a completion but the tendency is certainly there.

Anthony Williams (1989) writes convincingly of the benefits of action methods in psychodrama and relates them especially to the life of the family. He states:

1. Enactment changes the mode in which the family commonly expresses itself . . . Imagination and spontaneity take on concrete form and recursively feed into the family's concept of itself.

2. Action methods can be used as analogic representations of differences in the family. The method is capable of illustrating intangibles more clearly than most other techniques.
3. It dramatises roles and role perceptions . . . the transactional nature of family roles, for example, becomes clearer.
4. It can re-create the past and bring it vividly into the here and now, thus allowing the re-editing of family myths.
5. It can be used to enact fantasies of the future . . . unanticipated consequences of action can be made real.
6. The transactional and systemic meanings of family behaviour can be uncovered and elucidated in role analysis.
7. The family is enabled to act out rituals concerning rites of passage, or ways of marking differences this allows the family to make distinctions.

Although Williams relates these benefits to the work with families it is obvious that they are capable of universal application, revised according to the context in which the psychodramatist may be working.

There are many other beneficial attributions that can be discovered in the work of psychodrama but now let us consider some of the limitations of the method.

Primacy of group needs

The most obvious limitation is that individuals have to subsume their own personal needs for attention to the climate of the group as a whole and the awareness of the director. It has to be faced that directors vary a good deal in their skill and sensitivity and their ability to 'handle' a group. It is more difficult for individuals to challenge the director in the group setting, which in any case is likely to be more controlling of individuals than would be experienced in one-to-one therapy. So the individual is subject to the opportunities and creativity of the group, which will obviously vary from group to group, and this could be very limiting.

Preoccupation with conscious states

Psychodrama may be limited in its approach to that which is usually recognized as conscious states, unless the director has a special interest in the psychology of the unconscious, which, sometimes, is unlikely. The most obvious examples of unconscious material coming to play in the psychodrama setting is manifested by body posture, the disposition of characters in the scene, the management of furniture, and 'errors' of speech and description. For example, in one drama that I was conducting, the protagonist repeatedly mistook the role-play father for the role-play mother with much resultant confusion. In another a client 'forgot' to put a chair in the sitting room he would normally sit in. The situation was finally addressed as a significant part of the psychodrama because I, as the director, saw significance in what was happening and drew attention to it as therapeutic material to work with, rather than merely 'correcting' these pathological slips, as Freud (1975c) would have identified them.

The role of unconscious material

We know that unconscious material can 'leak' into consciousness during a role play, and this material may come from the protagonist or from other members of the group. It is in respect to the latter that we need to remain aware of its potentially disrupting influence. Powerful defensive feelings may come into play when the protagonist attempts to address very difficult, ambiguous and threatening issues from her life space. Insight is inhibited and rationalizing takes the place of a genuine emotional encounter. If the director is unaware of, or unable to confront, such an occurrence then the therapy is impaired.

Intrusion may come, too, from members of the group who unwittingly, prompted by unconscious anxiety, may become over-identified with the protagonist's situation and process and consequently introduce material that distorts the work of the protagonist. This is evident sometimes in demanding doubling. As mentioned in Chapter Two, Dean Elfthery had an expression for this: he would ask 'well whose psychodrama is this anyway?'

Time limitations

A more serious drawback, in my view, is the relatively short space of therapy time a psychodrama will occupy in a client's life. This is especially true if the psychodrama is only on offer as an occasional workshop, usually conducted at a weekend session. The situation is better if the psychodrama group is available on a weekly basis, each meeting lasting for two to three hours. But, like most group psychotherapy, it cannot compare with the amount of time and attention a client will receive in weekly, hour-long, individual psychotherapy sessions. Some clients need a lengthy individual therapeutic relationship.

The unstable arrangements that may go with the psychodrama group is another factor with which one must reckon. At one time I came across a psychodramatist, working sessionally for a large hospital, who would be asked to come to the ward to conduct a psychodrama. Once he had 'obliged' he was sent on his way, perhaps never to see those patients again. The psychodramatist concerned felt this keenly but still found himself falling in with such requests.

Suitability for psychodrama

Although I am of the opinion that psychodrama as a therapy should be available to all who wish to work in that mode, I am very aware that some clients, especially those in institutions where they are disempowered, might come to dread the performing and exposing character of psychodrama when they do not wish to participate. Even as a relatively experienced psychoanalytical psychotherapist, with a background as an actor and director and some professional broadcasting experience in radio and television, I can remember the feeling of anxiety that would invade me when it came to my turn to perform, even though I had volunteered to perform and I trusted the psychodrama directors. We should remember that the process is powerful and psychodrama may not be for everyone. It may not be the client's 'cup of tea'. The client should, as with every therapy, be informed and be given the chance to choose. This is not to say that the resistance should never be challenged, but rather that the client's refusal should be taken seriously, not being unduly pathologized through inappropriate interpretation.

Psychodrama is time consuming

Psychodrama certainly normally requires more than the one-and-a-half hours allocated to most group psychotherapies. It can be difficult to find time for it. Recently advising a therapist, who is proposing to work in a therapeutic community, I found myself suggesting that he ask for a whole afternoon – to allow for the pre-group meeting with his co-therapist, for time for the group to meet and select a protagonist and work and share, all this to be followed by time for him to debrief with his co-therapist.

The need for space and equipment

Another potential drawback for the psychodrama group is the need to provide generous space and equipment for the group to use towards therapeutic ends. A room for a sitting-down group with, say, eight people in it can be quite modest in its proportions. But the psychodrama group needs a room that is *at least* twenty feet square and it is very helpful to the group to be properly provided with elementary props together with material and lighting to enhance its work. None of this might be available to a small psychotherapy unit struggling with a lack of resources in an NHS setting, fraying at the edges as a result of economies.

This is a brief survey of some of the advantages and disadvantages of psychodrama as a therapy and as an approach to dealing with clients' needs. As far as emotional and mental states are concerned I think it is most effective when the client can be coherent and active in the process of 'telling her story'. Obviously conditions such as the presence of deep depression with all its accompanying loss of interest and energy may prove to be quite impervious to the work of the psychodramatist.

Sometimes people who suffer delusions, distorting reality in a serious way, may find that they cannot accept, or open themselves up to, the demands of a psychodrama group. The same may apply to persons who are seriously sociopathic and find the interventions of the group intolerable. But these states are often not *absolute* and sometimes clients, apparently falling into these categories, may wish to enter a psychodrama group in order to test the therapy, to discover if they can use the method. Frankly, unless there are very good reasons, this desire should not be resisted – rather, it should be encouraged. Often patients with such reservations will need quite a lot of time in a psychodrama group, observing and working in ancillary roles before daring to embrace the role of protagonist. So with permission from the group members, admission to the group should be conducted in a liberal non-exclusive manner.

In conclusion, it remains true that psychodrama appears to be no less valuable as a therapy than any other approach. I think the issue of choice is critical, and that it should be available to clients if they require it. Having said that, it then becomes obvious that its presence, character and quality must be known to clients if they are to make an informed choice.

Chapter 5

A diagrammatic description of psychodrama

'The Guests are met, the feast is set,
May'st hear the merry din.'

Samuel Taylor Coleridge
The Rime of the Ancient Mariner. Part 1.

In this chapter I wish to express my appreciation to Doreen Elefthery and to the late Dean of the International Foundation for Human Relations for providing me with the model of work from which this diagrammatic representation through words is drawn.

The aim is to give the reader, unfamiliar with the practise of psychodrama, a diagrammatic 'birds eye' view of the structure and movement that is central to the therapeutic procedure.

The five instruments

- The protagonist – who emerges from the group interaction.
- Auxiliary egos – extensions of the life space of the protagonist, drawn from the group by the protagonist.
- The group – members who come together to enact a psychodrama with the chosen protagonist.
- The director – the therapist who provides creative direction and maintains the boundaries of the group.
- The stage – a physical area wherein the protagonist and group can encounter the psychodramatic action in its past, present and future representations.

Psychic stages	The unconscious state;
	The pre-conscious state;
	The conscious state;
	The presence of new conscious experience and material.
Levels of action	Talking in the group;
	The emergence of the protagonist;
	The warm up;
	Moving into action;
	Closure in sharing.

In brief, a psychodrama may be summed up as having three major parts under which the above may be subsumed:

- *The warm-up period.* This is the period when the group and the therapist explore personal and group needs, sometimes through action, metaphorical and symbolic, until ready to move into dramatic activity with a protagonist.
- *Action.* A protagonist emerges and a psychodrama is performed under the direction of the psychodramatist, with members assisting the protagonist in enacting aspects of her life space, through the process of acting as auxiliary egos or through doubling.
- *Sharing and feedback; closure.* This is a time when group members have an opportunity to share with the protagonist their individual experience of the psychodrama from the viewpoint of participator or observer. This time is not used to extend the work of the protagonist – it is essentially a time of sharing by group members of *their own* experience within the closure.

Some notes

Freudian psychoanalysis as revealed in Freud's own case studies assumes the significance of family life, although contemporary psychoanalytical psychotherapists seem sometimes to have overlooked this historical fact.

Psychodrama supports the significance of social experience in the development of the personality. It is primarily an existential therapy, using an interactionist model, influenced by psychoanalytic concepts. *Thought and feeling*, from sources of family and social life, provide the route to *action*.

Psychodrama relates to the idea of catharsis, through which a new balanced view of life may be achieved, as being an important element of therapeutic experience. It is a group therapy introduced into the United States by Moreno (1957), relating to and influencing theories of group analysis in the UK, Foulkes (1957). It is able to work through the whole spectrum of time – past, present and future. As with the formal Greek tragic dramas, it works within the structure of time, place and person.

The director

The director is:

- directive;
- instigative;
- interpretative;
- empathic;
- self restraining;
- aware and responsive to both *tele* and *transference* feelings when manifested towards herself, to other individuals, to the group in parts, or to the group as a whole;
- is the instrument for leading the protagonist from *thought and feeling into action*.

Technique

Spontaneous creative expression within a carefully devised format. It is able to locate itself in any aspect of place through the process of improvisation and spontaneous action in the here and now. Sometimes free association will occur as part of the spontaneous activity.

Ethics

It is client centred and, although 'directed', it remains within the control of the client through a dialogue that seeks permission before enactment.

Confidentiality is held by the psychodrama director (no disclosure) but is realistically conditioned by the nature of the group membership. There can be no absolute expectation of confidentiality although most groups become respectful of its importance as an aspect of group life and culture.

The professional relationship

Earlier in this book I referred to Moreno's (1934) concept of *tele*. I acknowledge its importance and centrality to the practice of psychodrama. Indeed it is obvious to any psychodramatist that warmth, trust, empathy, unconditional regard and congruence (Rogers, 1969) are essential conditions for the effective use of the psychodramatic technique in psychotherapy. This view is very close to Moreno's notion of *tele*. Wilkins (1999) argues that there are no absolute conflicts between Moreno's position and Rogers'. I do not intend here to pursue this view but merely assert that psychodrama, to be effective, must rest upon strong feelings of confidence in the director and the support of the group. Thus it is essentially an emotional experience, albeit accompanied by cognitive insights. I am arguing that the protagonist moves more confidently and therapeutically into action when this condition of emotional connection is experienced. For many participants in the emerging psychodrama group there is much work to be done in establishing fully trusting relationships with the director and other members of the group before moving confidently into action.

Blatner (1988) understands psychodrama as a method firmly attached to existential therapy and, consequently, a humanistic perspective, where the values of the approach are firmly rooted in respect for human relationships and a belief in the possibility of change in response to insight and understanding. A number of authors, including William Schultz, Harold Mosak and Rudolf Dreikurs, Walter Kempler and Carl Rogers all acknowledge the place and influence of psychodrama within humanistic therapies of differing categories.

Understanding and accepting this view does not imply a rejection of the position that psychoanalytic psychodramatists might hold. The distanced, reserved viewpoint of the analyst in either traditional group psychotherapy or individual psychotherapy is not appropriate to the practice of psychodrama – so much is obvious. But the insights of the analytic position need not be lost. As Freud states, transference and its importance, which seems to excite the most difficulty for therapists of other disciplines, is *not* in the possession of psychoanalysis. Transference, as I have argued elsewhere, is a phenomenon that exists and is active in all human relationships in any human context, within and outwith psychoanalysis. Therefore it must be present within the psychodramatic context. As Yalom (1975) states, it is a matter of what you do about it.

Paul Wilkins (1997) gives us a good example of how he resolved what I would see as a transference experience within the mode of a psychodrama.

Scene 22 – a psychodrama performance (Paul Wilkins reporting)

I became aware that the process between us somehow reflected what he was attempting to resolve in the drama. My sense was of being silently requested for something I could not provide. At this I experienced a gut churning sense of inadequacy which I knew to be connected with the process as the psychodrama was unfolding in the way the protagonist desired. At a suitable moment I said to the protagonist, 'It's as if you wanted more from your father then he could offer and I sense I too am not giving you what you want.' The protagonist nodded vigorously, my gut churning sensation disappeared and the protagonist returned to the scene with vigour.

It is possible that Wilkins would not accept my understanding of what occurred as an example of transference resolution but I leave readers to interpret the material as they wish. I have no wish to split hairs. It is quite obvious, though, that both Paul and his client were moving from *thought into feeling and action.*

The existential model of psychotherapy does not, in principle, reject the concept. Indeed, it seems to me that 'tele' and 'transference' exist together in the psychodrama group as a creative tension when the protagonist finds the courage and energy to perform. Many other key psychoanalytic concepts, including the most influential of all Freudian assertions – the centrality of the unconscious in shaping the psychological destinies of men and women – remain present in the practice of psychodrama.

This short chapter has set out the basic structure of the psychodrama session and it has explained and illuminated the principal roles of the human participants. In the next chapter we shall encounter the therapeutic experience as it arises from this structure and methodology.

Chapter 6

From thought and feeling into action

'Lights, camera, action!'

In this chapter the diagrammatic headings are expanded and examined in closer detail as a working method. Let us return to the stages of work that have been outlined in the structure already described in Chapter 5.

The group meets and its members talk to each other and the director

At this stage the experienced director allows a free flow of feeling, ideas and information. At this stage her task is to listen and influence in an accommodating and supportive way. A good deal of thinking, with consequent talking, is going on. Confidence can only grow in the group as it explores its existence and begins to accept itself as a social organism. Its members have to *practise* acceptance and interest in each other as members of the group. Each member has to learn to listen, to pay attention to the expressed needs of other members of the group. Each member has to accommodate to sharing and waiting for the right moment to enter the group discussion. Each member has to deal with irrational feelings of attraction and dislike that might easily occur in the opening phases of the group.

Scene 23

A large room in a psychotherapy treatment centre. It is morning.

The second meeting of a psychodrama group. There are 10 members in the group, but at the first meeting only nine were present. Jane had sent her apologies; she had joined at the last moment and would not be coming until the second meeting. The group sat quietly waiting. Nothing had been said about the expected Jane. The group had been sitting in relative silence for five minutes, Jane was not present. Some members were very aware of her absence, others had 'forgotten' that she was supposed to be present. No chair had been put out for her so the group was in a closed circle. Slowly the door opened, those sitting facing it saw a small face peering anxiously in. It was Jane. She spoke. 'Oh I'm so sorry to disturb you, but is this the group? You know, the psychodrama group?'

The group was suddenly electrified. Three people immediately jumped up to welcome her. She came through the door swiftly and smoothly. She wore a silky flowing skirt that swished with energy as she came through the door. She ignored the men who were on their feet greeting her. She spotted a chair up against the wall and with entirely unexpected strength swung it upwards and forwards towards the group almost as if to attack it. She paused for a fraction of a moment and advanced determinedly towards David. 'Move up!' she cried. 'This is where I'm going to sit.' After much shoving about and adjustment of chairs and bodies Jane settled back into her chair. 'Terribly sorry about being late. Motorway in a terrible mess.' She glanced fondly at David. 'But anyway I'm here now, so thank goodness for that.'

The group met for about two years. Jane sat beside David throughout the entire time. He was quite entranced by her for some of that time. Some of the men in the group felt jealous of the attention she gave to David, especially in the early stages. Some resented her influence within the group, both with the men and the women. Others appeared quite indifferent to the David–Jane diad relationship.

What is most striking about the anecdote is how it describes an instant attraction that was acted upon within the therapy group. A group analyst would have probably been thinking in terms of Bion's (1961) theory of 'pairing', but for the psychodrama director, although aware of this phenomenon, it was an occurrence that would work itself out within the action of the group. As the director of the group she would have to work in such a way that neither Jane nor David unduly controlled the work of the other. This would be done through the work encouraged within the psychodrama action, as she acted as a dramatic director and within the sharing sessions the group would experience. The aim of the psychodramatist would be much the same as the group analyst, which would be for the group to take responsibility for itself as a group, where all the members contribute meaningfully and a 'pair' is neither encouraged nor left to do all the work, producing magical solutions to problems while others look on, passive, distanced, lethargic or even just enjoying the 'show'.

From thought and feeling into action

Of course the director can expedite the process of meeting and getting to know that has to take place. There are a whole number of games and activities that will accelerate the socializing and learning process. One of my favourites is to invite a new group to play the 'magic shop' game, with myself in the role of awkward shopkeeper. This game not only reveals a good deal about the aspirations and character of the players but accustoms the group to the idea of playing in fantasy. It is regressive, in a benign sense of the word. It takes players back to the playground and the world of childhood wishes. The game is simple enough. The shopkeeper in the magic shop has a stock of attributes at her disposal. The individual customers come to trade with her. But barter is the name of the game and the individual has to persuade the shopkeeper to accept one human attribution in exchange for another. Played imaginatively the possibilities of the exchange are almost endless. In one game, a few years ago, playing the shopkeeper I insisted I had very little *tolerance* in stock but I was anxious to unload a lot of *sentimentality*. The resulting confusion and frustration opened up a lot of issues and encouraged members of the group to express openly their ideas and feelings about the way they were being manipulated by an apparently depriving and contriving shopkeeper. Playing shopkeeper and customer opens up a world of meaning relating to the roles we play in our lives and the symbolic meaning of the attributes we value as individuals. The world of dramatherapy has a host of such imaginative games at the disposal of players and I am grateful for my training as a dramatherapist because it equipped me with a rich repertoire of 'warm-up' activities. Sue Jennings (1973) places a good deal of stress on the place of improvisation as a creative medium for emotional learning and also points to the human need to play in order to achieve creativity in life.

And so the group meets and talks. But they are talking to some purpose. The aim of the group is to be a therapeutic milieu from which individuals may emerge to identify difficulties and confusions, problems and pain in their lives and to take some action to highlight the dilemma, explore its nature and reach for possible resolution.

The protagonist emerges

This is simply the person who chooses to occupy the psychodramatic stage with the permission, approval and support of the director and the rest of the group. The task of the protagonist is to 'live in the present' (Schutzenberger, 1975). He brings the history of his behaviour into the present and examines it critically through the medium of role play and psychodramatic invention. The protagonist has at his disposal Moreno's

(1972) notion of the 'social atom' – all the significant relationships that an individual has at any given time, these relationships being defined by interaction.

Scene 24

The psychodrama group. A training group meeting in a psychotherapy centre.

The group has been talking for about 15 minutes. John has already made a bid for attention. He wants to work on his relationship with his dead father. Mary has made one or two remarks but appears to be hanging back, deferring to John. The group is becoming aware of this.

Harry: 'Was it always like this for you, Sue, when you were a kid?'

Mary: 'Well not always, it wasn't so bad when my brother left school and went to work. Of course I was still at the girl's grammar school. There are four years between us. But before that it was terrible. I was terrified of him. And mum was no help; none at all.'

John: 'I know exactly what you mean. My mother was and still is absolutely useless if you want a bit of support. It's always 'Oh don't upset me, I can't bear to hear it' and so on.'

He is still bidding for attention, albeit without conscious intent.

Harry (ignoring John's intervention): 'Well Mary why don't you do some work about this?'

Director: 'Yes Mary, why not.'

(Mary looks doubtful but gives the director a brief nod.)

Director: 'Harry, change places with me, let me sit next to Mary. Is that OK, Mary?'

(Mary smiles at him and nods again.)

There is a slight sigh of awareness and satisfaction by the rest of the group and John notes the director's intervention and smiles too, directly at Mary, as if to say that it is OK by him. Harry looks pleased. His encouragement and intervention have worked.

The protagonist emerges from this interplay within the group, subtly supported by the director and finally confirmed between the protagonist and the director together. Then follows a psychotherapeutic dialogue in which the director takes the lead, carefully helping the protagonist to outline and unravel her story, inviting her to move from the first position of feeling and talking to the next position of feeling and acting.

This is a critical dialogue for the director is going to move the protagonist from the past to the 'here and now' where attitudes and experiences are going to be confronted with new energy that flows from improvisation and spontaneity.

This is not easily done. It has to be borne in mind that many protagonists have been harbouring material of an undermining character in their lives for many years. The protagonist has probably sought all kinds of means to avoid confronting, or reliving the pain of the past. She has probably displaced it, distracted herself, substituted for it with fantasy, or a contrived loss of memory. She may have focused in an obsessive way on the future, avoiding at all costs the relationships and her realities as experienced in her present, which relate to the past. Given these possibilities then it should not be surprising to us that the protagonist is going to struggle to bring her focus into the 'here and now'. In the instance quoted, Mary was going to revisit the past and the sexual and emotional abuse practised by her older brother. The therapeutic dialogue between Mary and the director is the beginning of the psychodramatic frame; once Mary agrees to enter the frame then she is committing herself to continuing a journey the end of which she cannot forecast with any certainty. Mary has moved through the stages of thought and feeling and is now going to enter the stage of dramatic action.

The issue of who shall become the protagonist is sometimes a central experience for the psychodrama group. I have been in groups where it is assumed that every one had to 'have a chance'. Then there is a kind of deferment between members of the group, until some sort of pecking order is worked out to the satisfaction of the group. This is a dynamic process and it is up to the director to decide whether to challenge it or not. In the case of Vladimir (Scene 12, pp. 25–6) I decided to intervene to give him another chance to work against the resistance he was feeling towards exploring his feelings towards his wife, which went beyond anger. It meant asking the group for permission to do this, thus displacing the natural expectations of the group. It was almost certain that some other member of the group would have come to the session that day expecting to be the protagonist. It is impossible to decide, in advance of the event, what to do when circumstances present themselves that call for the director to intervene in the internal dynamics of the group. But certainly the time will come. So it is well to be prepared.

I believe that the presence of a person in a psychodrama group implies that the person concerned wants at some point to become the protagonist. Sometimes it is far from obvious and most directors have experienced the group member, who whilst keen to work for others as an auxiliary, or is active in doubling and sharing, holds back from personal performance. Moreno too insisted that at points in a psychodrama the group itself becomes the protagonist. I believe this happens through collective identification with the protagonist. So the reluctant member may indeed be working for herself, whilst at the same time avoiding the direct confrontation that the protagonist role calls for. Should the director do anything about this? Well it seems likely that the usual requirement is for the director to address the issue in an open and challenging way. The advice, however, is not to be threatening or manipulative, in a coercive way. What makes this an imperative is that the group itself will have already noticed what is happening and may well be waiting for the director to open up the issue.

The group may well be angry with this non-performing member who is active on the scene but without that direct, open commitment to action that the rest of members are offering each other. They may interpret the behaviour as voyeuristic. Indeed it may well be so. There is, within virtually all human beings, a desire to experience emotional gratification through witnessing the emotions of others, whether they be painful or pleasurable. A good deal of excitement is experienced in such situations and the onlooker is sometimes a figure that arouses anxiety, confusion and anger. The act of becoming the protagonist is an act of identification with the mores of the group, which is valued by the membership, establishing the person as having entered the group in a meaningful way. The individual should regard it as an important aspect of the process of confirmation of group membership. Equally important is the presence of the group member who, hungry for attention, care, interest and help, constantly asks for the protagonist role.

Scene 25

A large open space in a conference centre in the north of England. A conference of therapists some years ago. A distinguished psychodramatist has been asked to make a contribution to the work of the conference. He has been given the whole membership of the conference to work with, other than those who choose not to come to this session. The psychodramatist states that he intends to offer an opportunity to any member of the conference to perform a psychodrama. John, my companion, an experienced psychotherapist, looks at me quizzically. I feel a wave of anxiety go through me. What is going to happen? There are some 70 people present, many of us strangers to each other. There is a pause as the psychodramatist announces his intention. The group is sitting in a double circle. One circle inside the other. A long moment stretches into a longer one. The psychodramatist, who is standing more or less in the centre of the inner circle, looks around with an encouraging half smile. He too is waiting. There is a shuffling of bodies, one or two incoherent whispers are heard, but not understood. The group members are innocent of this approach and are instinctively going into a defensive posture. The psychodramatist repeats his offer. This does it! A young woman, from the outer circle, is struggling to her feet and speaking to the therapist. She is volunteering to work. John looks at me with an expression of concern on his face. We both know this young woman. She is in training to become a psychotherapist but the training is only a slightly disguised way of experiencing therapy as a patient. Her name is Marion and Marion is well known locally for her interventions that seek to place her in the role of need. John is dismayed. I feel disturbed too, but also curious. Will the psychodramatist take this offer at its face value? I wait to see how it will be resolved.

Over an hour later Marion is deeply involved with a painful, exposing psychodrama. The psychodramatist seems happy to continue and has drawn members of the audience into the performance in the roles of auxiliary figures. Marion herself cooperates happily with the director, seeming unaware of any difficulty or ethical problem in her performance situation. John and I have withdrawn to the outer edges of the group in an act of unconscious disassociation. We are disturbed by the hazard of this enterprise where there is no protection for the protagonist in respect of future work or in respect of confidentiality and further support from the group. I am reminded of reports of large audience psychodramas that were carried out by Moreno in a public theatre in the early days of the development of the therapy and the distaste I felt for it then and still do now.

So the over-eager protagonist may seduce the eager director. I can only imagine the director in this case wanted to satisfy the organizers, who were looking to witness the expertise of this well-known and publicized psychodramatist, who took up the offer, the first to come to hand, from eager Marion. And it should not be overlooked that the large audience group was looking for action too. Another pressure on the visiting director and, of course, on Marion.

The psychodramatist going into a stranger situation must be prepared for all sorts of experiences arising from the pathology or expectations of the group encountered. Some years ago, running a workshop, part lecture, part action, with a sophisticated group of professionals doing an advanced degree in psychotherapy studies in a university, I encountered a group member who felt and expressed acute anxiety at the probability of the open examination of any emotion in the group, especially that concerned with loss and bereavment, by another group member. This was in circumstances where I had carefully devised a work format demonstrating some of the main techniques of psychodrama without involving any individual in a personal psychodrama to any depth. I invited anyone in the group to 'warm up' a significant figure from their life. A young personable man offered to 'warm up' his father who had died some months ago. I felt well aware of the significance of this choice but felt I could handle it satisfactorily. But as soon as the decision was made to work with him the young woman became distressed and virtually brought the workshop to a standstill. She could not tolerate the idea of his working in this kind of way, addressing his dead father. I tried to reassure her by reminding her that we all have conversations with figures in our lives who are dead or missing, living as they do as introjected figures in our psyche. But such was the force of her intervention I felt I had no option but to abandon the exercise and deal in the 'here and now' with her intervention within the limits of the lecture/workshop. Psychotherapy is a difficult, if not dangerous profession and psychodramatists in particular are subject to very vivid projections that sometimes need to be openly addressed and worked with as they occur.

The warm up

I have always liked this expression. It suggests to me the stimulation of psychic energy. A sense of engagement. Becoming a part of a process in an emotional manner, investing in a process. Anne Schutzenberger (1975) literally describes the warm up as 'breaking the ice', 'getting to know one another'. Another way of interpreting the expression is to see it as the necessary precursor of moving into the psychodrama. A group will often want to start its session by looking back at the previous sessions, reflecting upon subsequent feelings and other outcomes.

The 'warm up' is an integral part of the psychodrama ritual. Rituals hold great value to the group; rituals are a way of maintaining customary, valued and understood procedures that contain value for the group members. Sometimes the rituals are very powerful and withstand any attempts to change them. But in psychodrama it is rarely so. The rituals are generally more like habits – good therapeutic habits that are valued by the group.

When the protagonist has emerged then another stage of 'warm up' is entered into. The protagonist is usually invited to bring to the psychodramatic stage significant figures of the past and present. Members of the group, auxiliaries, are chosen by the protagonist to perform the role of these figures and they need to be informed concerning the figure to be played. This is quite a complicated business because as well as pragmatic information the auxiliary wants to know the emotional quality of the person she is playing. It is this description, through a dramatic dialogue, that constitutes an important aspect of 'warm up' for the auxiliary and for the protagonist offering the information. The most frequently used 'warm up' technique used for this purpose by the protagonist is the 'role reversal' technique. The process is illuminating not only to the auxiliary playing the role but also to the director and the audience and, not least, the protagonist.

Scene 26

Harry is standing behind an auxiliary who is portraying his dead mother. He stands with his hands on the shoulders of the auxiliary and starts to speak for his mother.

Harry: 'My name is Amy. I am . . . no, no, I was Harry's mother when I was . . .'

There is a long pause. Harry's eyes are filling with tears. He is now not so much as touching the auxiliary performer as gripping her shoulders.

Harry (starts to talk again now 'out of role'): 'I didn't think I would cry like this. What am I crying for?'

He looks appealingly to the director. The director waits for a moment or two and the auxiliary finds her voice.

The auxiliary, playing Amy, speaks: 'Harry was my first and my favourite. He must miss me a good deal, it was awful parting from him.'

Harry now finds the strength to continue.

Harry (in role reversal now with his mother): 'I didn't want to die. It was a shame I was only 66. Silly to die at that age. I had so much to live for. Well there was Harry and Sally, the kids, then there was Jim, my husband, a lovely fellow, I really loved him. Then along came the stupid old cancer, and that was that. I had to go.'

Harry is now speaking freely without reserve. He is able to speak fluently for his mother.

In a warm up like this, the auxiliary, the director and the group, are offered intimate and revealing information, notably about the quality and depth of Harry's feelings towards his mother, but they are given a picture, too, of his mother's place in the family, as seen by Harry.

Moving into action

Although, in a sense, it can be said a psychodrama commences with the coming together of the group, for most people the drama starts after the protagonist emerges and after the setting up of the scene. Both the audience and the protagonist are now at the point of 'action' or 'doing'. This action may be very physical or it may be primarily verbal; usually, of course, it is a mixture of both. The dramatic reality is that action starts when a relationship is encountered on the stage and the quality and content of that relationship is behaved by the protagonist and the supporting auxiliary performers. So action is the drama. It may have the quality of absolute stillness. The director may well ask the protagonist to take up a position that reflects, in a living sculpture, the essence of the relationship with another person. This is 'action'. A dramatic cameo is devised and presented. To be active the stage does not have to be full of people running around, as if in a Whitehall farce.

Scene 27

A psychodrama performance in a therapeutic community. The protagonist is discovered sitting in an arm chair beside which there is a coffee table. On the coffee table is a mock telephone. The protagonist is waiting in silence for the telephone to ring. She sits for what seems an interminable period of silence, waiting. She sits still, attentive and alert, not slumped in the chair but upright.

The director gives a cue: 'OK the phone is ringing. Listen – the phone is ringing, you can hear it.' The protagonist sits staring at the phone without moving.

The director speaks again: 'It is still ringing, you can hear it.'

The protagonist leans forward, picks up the phone and listens carefully for a moment. There is no expression on her face. She looks quite blank but very attentive to a voice at the other end of the phone, which no one else hears. Then she puts the phone down, quietly and carefully and flops back into the chair.

Soon she will speak. The group and the director are patient and let her work at her own pace.

This scene was full of action – emotional action that held the audience in suspense. We have all seen similar scenes of emotional action in the theatre and in our everyday lives we are familiar with its intensity. It is rich in meaning.

Scene 28

The same group as above. A protagonist has been complaining of feeling trapped by her family. She is a mother to three growing-up young people. But she is very passive in her telling. She whines out her complaint. There is little energy present. The director decided to symbolize her situation in a physical way. The protagonist is sitting in an armchair near the sitting-room fire. The young people are present, all played by auxiliary egos.

The director says to the players: 'Well, mother is going to try to get out of her chair. You must try to stop her. No talking.'

The players stand around the chair and mother makes a feeble attempt to leave the chair. The young people prevent her by holding her down in the chair, she wriggles rather than struggles.

The director says: 'Come on mother, try a bit harder.'

The auxiliary players are now looking a bit embarrassed. The protagonist tries again, this time with a little more effort, but is easily defeated. One of the young people, a lively looking boy is now sitting on her lap.

The director intervenes again. Now he calls upon his co-director to take the place of the protagonist in the chair and he invites the protagonist to stand beside him and watch a replay of the scene. Nothing is said but the protagonist watches with interest and finally speaks.

Protagonist: 'Well it rather looks as if I don't want to leave that chair doesn't it.'

Director: 'But we do see who you would like to have on your lap, don't we! He looks very comfortable!'

Here there is plenty of physical action but the dramatic 'action' lies in the emotional quality of the symbolic activity and its implied meaning, which is shared by everyone present.

Sometimes it is difficult for the protagonist to move into action. The protagonist appears to be stuck; she becomes emotionally stupid, unable to think or feel her way forward into the drama. This is usually an instance of 'resistance'. Here I am referring to a psychoanalytic concept where the client experiences a powerful controlling intervention from the unconscious that inhibits the revelation of disturbing material. In psychodrama it is as if the ability to be spontaneous and improvisatory is lost, which it clearly is, when the protagonist behaves in such a manner, having apparently lost the creative ability to work therapeutically. Sometimes this means the protagonist is held in a role from which she finds it impossible to shift.

There are a number of reasons advanced in psychodramatic theory to account for this state of being. The most apparent feeling is usually that of anxiety in the protagonist. But this tells us very little. Is the anxiety the cause of the loss of spontaneity or merely a product of the loss of creativity? Chicken or egg dilemma. Which comes first? Moreno (1934) would probably have thought that the anxiety arises from the loss of spontaneity, the loss of creative resources. But this does not answer the question as to why this loss should occur. The psychoanalytical approach is helpful here because this approach will take us back to the first position of defence within the psyche. If the material being approached is too threatening to the client then a defence will be mounted to avoid exposure. Hence the stuckness and 'stupidity' is being unable to think or feel effectively.

So the director is then faced with a problem: how to respond. The first rule is that the director must avoid being put into the position of conflict with the protagonist. If this should happen then the 'working alliance' of the director and protagonist is threatened. The notion of 'working alliance' is again drawn from psychoanalytic thought. It was a response to trying to identify the quality of the relationship between therapist and patient that was not vested in 'transference'. The essential quality being identified is the obvious desire of the therapist and the patient to work together towards a therapeutic end in a joint enterprise. An experience of benign collaboration. Resistance in the protagonist puts this alliance at risk. So the director has to resist any compulsion in herself to prematurely pressure the protagonist into giving up the resistance.

In practice it is usually necessary for the director to manoeuvre and negotiate with the protagonist to move into channels of expression that are acceptable to the protagonist. In other words it is necessary for the director to work *with* the resistance rather than *against* it in the first instance. Having said this, however, it must be borne in mind that there are no universal panaceas to guide us in the role of director. What I have written must be interpreted in relation to the actual relationship we have with our protagonist when we are in the directorial role. The quality of 'tele' and transference within the therapeutic relationship will be the guide to action.

Scene 29

Malcolm was sitting on a bus on the way to the hospital. Malcolm was dreading this day. He had agreed to work in psychodrama for the first time. This agreement had been forthcoming from him in the previous session with his group. Now the time had come. The bus stopped. He got off and turned into the drive of the hospital. His legs were leaden. How would he manage? He was dull and heavy. Only anxiety filled the space of his thinking and feeling.

He should never have agreed to this psychodrama business. He had watched others. But their sensitivity, insight and skill only made him feel more clumsy and stupid. He liked Helen the director, but she could push you on! Would she push him on? Would she? He dreaded the thought.

He was late for the group as he walked into the clinic. They were sitting waiting for him. His chair had been put out for him. Mary smiled at him encouragingly as he sat down. She was a good soul. Helen greeted him. There was silence. It was a strained, awkward affair. He felt they were all looking at him. He stared at the ground to avoid the pressure. But it did not go away. Helen spoke quietly to him.

Director: 'Do you want to work Malcolm?'

Malcolm: 'I don't know.'

There was another silence.

Malcolm: 'I can't think of anything, nothing.' *(And then with emphasis)*: 'Nothing!' *(More silence.)*

Malcolm: 'Can't get up and act. You know, not like the others.'

Director: 'Yes I know. Well shall we just talk?'

Malcolm: 'Yes, if you like.'

Director: 'No not as I like. But as you like Malcolm. What do you think?'

Malcolm: 'Ok. Yeah, that's OK. I can talk but I can't act no part, I surely can't.'

But he knows his mind is clearing, the dullness is lifting, he is beginning to feel warm towards Helen, she is going to help him. The fear of overwhelming control and manipulation is clearing.

Closure in sharing

The closure of a psychodrama comes in a number of stages. There is usually a natural, dramatic closure. The director 'tracking' the drama as it unfolds is usually in a position to know when this is going to occur. The director may well help a protagonist to recognize that the time is coming when the action on stage is coming to an end. The ending on stage should mirror the opening. The auxiliaries are asked simply to go back to the group circle, holding themselves 'in role'. The protagonist is left on the stage with the director and co-therapist and sets about removing the set, its props and furniture. This also includes de-roling symbolic objects that have been used to represent significant parts of the protagonist's life. An example would be where a tatty old paperback novel has been used to represent an important diary. An object of much significance and an essential aid to the action. Here the protagonist would simply de-role by stating the obvious:

Protagonist: 'This is a paperback novel, not my diary.'

A reader might think such a simple, obvious, statement is superfluous, but it must be remembered that the protagonist is moving from one reality to another and these rituals are necessary *rites of passage* from one state of being to another. So the simple statement of an obvious reality makes the passage clearer and easier.

When the stage is clear the protagonist moves off and away from it into the group. At this point she is probably feeling 'full' of material. She needs time to process the material inside herself. So from now on she sits and listens and the group allow her this space. No responses are required of her at all.

The auxiliaries now receive attention from the director. Playing an auxiliary is a special experience. More will be said about this in a later chapter.

At this point the director simply asks the auxiliary to de-role in the following manner.

John (an auxiliary who has played Fred, the protagonist's brother): 'I am not Fred, I am John.'

Director: 'Well, John, how did it feel when you were playing Fred? Can you describe your feelings as John first for us?'

John responds as well as he can.

Director: 'Now you are out of role, John, perhaps you can tell us what it was like for you to play Fred and perhaps you could share with us all any thoughts, feelings and memories that my have been stirred up for you.'

Readers will recall how in Scene 5 I described the reaction of an auxiliary who was called upon by members of the group to repeatedly play 'macho' punitive male roles and his feelings concerning this.

When the deroling is complete the rest of the group contribute. Their purpose is to share their *own* life experiences in a supportive way with the protagonist. Not to comment or extend the drama they have just seen. When the last one has finished it was always my practice, part of the ritual, to thank everyone who had contributed to the psychodrama, refer to any special needs expressed, thank the protagonist, and formally declare the session closed.

In the instance I have quoted, however, it needs to be borne in mind that in an ongoing group this closure is merely to point towards further psychodramas which are to come. Who knows – the protagonist may well come back to the material again from another perspective. Shared material will certainly come through to the full production of a psychodrama. The life of the group is merely suspended by the closure until it meets again.

CHAPTER 7

The art of psychodrama

The director

> 'The best actors in the world, either for tragedy, comedy, history, pastoral, pastoral-comical, historical-pastoral, tragical historical, tragical-comical-historical-pastoral, scene individable or poem unlimited.'
>
> Shakespeare. *Hamlet*, Act 2, Scene 2

In this chapter I shall be discussing what makes a director effective, not only as a psychotherapist but also as a skilful drama director. This discussion will lead us into thinking about the remainder of the group, their performance as an *audience*, but especially as a *performing audience* and then on to the role of the protagonist in her relationship with the director. All the members of the group, including the director, have to be able to 'play many parts' and yet it will be unlikely that any of them, with the possible exception of the director, have received any dramatic training. Does this matter? Well, clearly not very much, otherwise few psychodrama groups would have come into being.

The first requirement of the psychodrama director is that she has been properly trained as a psychotherapist and within that training has become a competent director. Another requirement of the director is that she be the most experienced client in the group. Her own training will have thoroughly inducted her into the role of client group member. Then she may know, in the most profound sense, the position of the client in the group. It is the equivalent of training therapy for the psychoanalytic psychotherapist or psychoanalyst. Without this experience the director is invalidated from the role of psychodramatist. A further requirement is that the director is motivated to be a psychodramatist for reasons of concern, caring and respect for other human beings in *their* struggle to live with *others* in their lives, whatever their difficulties, failure or success. The director has to have a moral base from which to work, which will inform her ethically, socially and psychologically in her relationships with her client group members. Without a moral base the work becomes empty and meaningless. This does not mean that psychodramatists have to subscribe to and share a common exclusive religious belief, humanistic credo or philosophical position. On the contrary, such a requirement would be restrictive and discriminative in its effects and finally destructive to our clients.

The director as a leader

There is sometimes an attempt made to persuade trainees that they should attach themselves to Moreno's charismatic personality and develop and respond to what today we would describe as a 'cult of the personality'. Freud, too, invited attachment in this way and actually created a group of supporters, who faithfully, unquestioningly, followed him. He rewarded them by membership of a secret inner circle whose identity was known by the possession of a special ring. There were unfortunate consequences, which encouraged rivalry and splitting. The consequences remain with us to this day. In our present time such a following would be regarded as an unhappy and destructive feature of any ideology, especially that which is so closely tied up with the nature of humanity, with which the theory and practice of psychodrama psychotherapy must be associated. Thus the most appropriate leadership style of our time is that of the democratic, participating leader who is open to suggestion, who is influenced by thought and feeling from her group; one who negotiates and learns from both clients and peers and is unthreatened by the excellence of others.

The moral director

It is true that Moreno strove to create a complete philosophy of life to which some were attracted, others not. His own view was that his most important text was *The Words of the Father* (1941). It was written and published in German at a very early stage in his career, as he states in his autobiography. Zerka Moreno, who was involved in the editing of a later version, published in English, was immediately in sympathy with this exposition. The book outlines and celebrates what may be described as an agnostic religion, where he places each and every individual as a creator within the dynamic configuration of the group, which is invested with almost superhuman creative power. Coming as it did in the early 20th century, the effect of this exhortation was to alienate the scientific attitude of many professionals working in the field of human relationships – especially the emerging psychologists, both academic and clinical, in America at this time. This was largely true of the response from medical men and women. We need to remember that modern psychiatry was in its infancy and striving for scientific recognition. Moreno's contribution seemed to confuse rather than enlighten. It is not for me to evaluate the strength of his philosophy here but simply to reiterate, in sympathy with Moreno, that psychotherapy has to be rooted in a moral framework and needs to be associated with a deep and profound humanism, respect being the key virtue. I remember recoiling in horror when a group analyst once stated, in a private conversation with me, that the insights of group analysis could be used effectively in the management of any group of people, irrespective of their social and moral condition. I immediately thought of the abuse of human groups that took place in Nazi death camps and in the Soviet Gulag. The British Psychodrama Association recognizes the need for an ethical code of behaviour and sets out a series of ethical statements to which all members and qualifying psychodramatists are expected to subscribe. This is common psychotherapeutic practice shared by all affiliates to the UKCP. It is obvious that these ethical statements, limited as they are, need to be incorporated into the therapist's personal moral stance, especially as it impinges upon her work as a therapist.

The director as artist

I have frequently taken part in discussion as to what part flair, artistry and talent play in the role of the psychodrama director. At one point in my life I was an untrained actor. Later on I trained as a director and drama teacher and taught secondary school children in a large comprehensive school in London. At another point I became a lecturer in drama, training drama teachers. I was also running, concurrently, a youth theatre in cooperation with a professional theatre in the north of England. In all these activities I was exploring my own creativity, discovering the possibilities of invention and performance. I think many psychodrama directors will share a similar background. I do not think for a moment that this kind of experience is necessary to become a successful psychodramatist, but it certainly helps. In a sense we are all actors but some of us are better than others at the art. And we also need to recognize that the director has a special brief to direct – that is to shape and organize the performance – not only therapeutically but in the aesthetic context of drama. In this respect the actors, including the protagonist, are relieved of what would otherwise be a demanding responsibility.

A psychodrama trainer, a Fellow of the American Society of Group Psychotherapy and Psychodrama, with whom I worked for many years, had come out of the background of work as an actress, a member of a distinguished theatre company. This was manifest in her work. The creative spirit was very evident and active in her when she was directing, co-directing or working as an auxiliary.

The essence of good drama lies in control. The actor strives to always be in control of his body and mind in performance. The training process in the actor strives to develop two apparently contradictory elements of the personality. Firstly are the qualities of control, especially of voice, body and the imagination in performance. Then there is the paradoxical need to encourage spontaneity in performance, enabling the actor to be free and creative. But these experiences are not contradictory; rather, they are complementary and, importantly, are subject to advancement and refinement. The psychodrama director, leading a training group, watching new embryonic directors performing, will encourage all of them equally. But at the same time the director will recognize talent when she sees it and this quality is often integral to a particular member of the group. As human beings we are all equal in value but we are certainly not all equal in talents. Some trainee directors have a natural 'feel' for direction; it is obvious in the dynamic, fluid competent and confident way they work, and this should be recognized by the training director. The problem the trainer has to resolve is how to praise and encourage without seeming to diminish the accomplishments of the rest of the group. Not for a moment should we lose sight of the importance of the director in the work of the group. Some of that importance is attached very firmly to her psychotherapeutic skill but some of it, quite properly, will rest in the director's artistic ability, her qualities as an artist and her ability to teach others.

The director as strong woman

A very important aspect of the director is her strength. Strength is not about her control in the sense of domination. This strength is shown in her ability to stand closely with the protagonist in the drama and at the same time remain at sufficient distance to be able to exercise therapeutic and artistic control. The artistic element is to do with assisting the protagonist in her performance and helping the protagonist to find a voice to express her feelings. This may even take some prompting and rehearsal. A strong director expands the possibilities of the group, the protagonist and the performance. As far as the therapeutic element is concerned, then, the strength of the director is discovered in her ability to enter where others may well fail to go, in the pursuit of truth, or paradoxically, to hold back and bear the distress of confusion when others might rush in to try be rid of confusion and ambivalence, finding both intolerable.

Scene 30

An outpatient group in an NHS psychotherapy centre. A psychodrama is proceeding. Jim the protagonist is speaking very quietly. There have already been several 'doubles' from the audience pointing out the significance of the virtual whispering. Jim appears to be keeping things to himself. Each time he is prompted he looks rather helplessly at the director for some help. The director is faced with two powerful aspects of performance. First the interpretation of the group who feel cut off, removed from Jim's dialogue, and the technical problem of dealing with Jim's very quiet voice and lack of projection.

Director (addressing her co-therapist): 'Harry, please stand with Jim and let us hear through you his responses, clearly, out loud for all to hear.'

And so the psychodrama proceeds, with both concerns addressed. The director would probably have been aware, too, how the small, whispering voice can dominate a scene. We are all forced to listen, to strain to catch the last word. It is often a source of manipulative control.

The safe director

Another evidence of strength is the ability of the director to maintain proper therapeutic boundaries, whilst at the same time remaining a flexible responsive director and human being. Both these functions need to be respected. They are at the heart of good psychodramatic performance. The psychodrama group comes into being at the behest of the director and the conditions of therapeutic performance are determined by her understanding, guidance and presence. Often the director has to address the reluctance to start the group, or address the late coming of one or two members, or it can be the reluctance to finish a group. Sometimes trainees in residential training groups, where time is very negotiable and the day may only be structured around meal times, might lose sight of the realities of other people's lives where time is constricted and bound around with family responsibilities. Nothing is more distracting and worrying when a director loses sight of the boundaries of a contract and the group continues to work beyond the agreed times of meeting. These may seem pedantic points of reference but the strength of these boundaries is a vital component of the therapeutic matrix and a measure of the director's competence and safety as a therapist.

The director as the memory

I have already mentioned 'tracking' as a skill and requirement of the psychodramatist. Keeping a record of the movement of the psychodrama from its very beginnings to its eventual performance and conclusion is a necessary attribute of the director. The protagonist often appears to lose this thread of continuity and needs reminding, through sensitive doubling, flashback work, or reflection, in order to remain coherently focused on the work in hand.

Scene 31

A therapeutic community within the NHS. It is late in the afternoon in the large group room. A psychodrama is moving towards its end. It has been a long hard struggle for Jennie and she has been working in the drama for nearly two hours. Now she is sitting alone in the setting of her sitting room at home, alone. She is ruminating in front of the fire.

Jennie: 'God knows what my daughter would think about all this. What a mother! God what a mess it has all been! Goodness knows what Carol thinks of me. Well at least I got that man out of my life, the sod! Ten years of misery, just thinking about it all the time and drinking myself silly. Poor old Carol.'

She pauses.

Director: 'But Jennie that is where you started, remember, with your daughter Carol. When we used the "empty chair" to bring her here to be with you. Right at the beginning. Why not bring her back and have a chat before we close the psychodrama.'

Jennie looks at the director with some surprise and then remembers too that the closure is approaching.

Jennie: 'Yeah, of course, I forgot all about that. How daft of me. It sounds like a good idea. But not the empty chair. Can I have someone to help me? What about you, Fatimah? It don't matter that you're an Indian – you look just like Carol, you remind me of her, such a pretty face.'

Fatimah smiles, pleased with having been described as having a pretty face, and comes into the acting area. The psychodrama proceeds.

This is just one example of the director being the memory of the group. This function is vital and is expected by the group either consciously or unconsciously. Members will expect the director to know and carry the memories of performance from one group meeting to another. Or, as in the example given, from one stage of the psychodrama to another.

The director as interpreter and analyst

This is central to the relationship of the director to the group and the protagonist. Psychodrama as a therapy is built around the notion of human beings learning to play roles. The assumption is that we are largely creatures of social construct and Moreno (1946) explored and elaborated this theory upon which the therapy of psychodrama depends. I shall say more about this in considering the place of the protagonist and group in the psychodramatic process. Psychodrama tends to be concerned with problems and difficulties in a specific sense. Clients coming to the psychodrama group may well have a sense of grievance or oppression arising from dysfunctional relationships which distorts the playing of a personal, albeit learned, role. As a director and as a patient I have been familiar with this process and looked to the work of the psychodrama group as a means of relieving the contradictions and tensions of the situation. But – and this is an important 'but' – sometimes the expressed problem is masking another, perhaps more difficult problem, which is being avoided. This masking process is known to us all. It is recalled in the following case.

This account comes from my individual practice as an psychoanalytic psychotherapist. A recent client was recalling how his young son of six years became 'mother's little helper' when a new baby was born – a very well-defined role. He would run and carry for his mother at her behest, without hesitation; he appeared to get satisfaction from his helping hands. He did not appear to have a problem. He was being rewarded by his mother's smiles and appreciation and this pleased him. But what was being masked of course was his jealousy of the new baby, the 'damned baby'. He could not articulate any of this jealousy, or his sense of being pushed out by the attention the baby was receiving from mother and, for that matter, father. Neither parent understood their son's problem in this way. His displacement was not known to him in any conscious sense. He had a general sense of anxiety, as a six-year-old child, which was relieved to some extent by being mother's little helper. But he was not her baby. There was some satisfaction, too, in standing between his mother and father in this self-appointed role but it didn't get rid of the problem of the 'damned baby'. It was to surface again much later in the little boy's life, in his adult relationship with women, where he lived in a continual fear of disappointing them, failing their emotional needs, and finally meeting emotional rejection, as they chose someone else to replace him.

The task of the psychodrama, then, was to have him remember the good moments of serving mother when he was a young boy, but in the here and now to interpret the feelings in a different way. Not to deny the pleasure of being 'mother's little boy', but rather to link these early Oedipal feelings, combined with the jealousy felt and repressed towards his baby sister, with his current state of thinking and feeling about women.

The director as psychologist

So the director of a psychodrama group needs the psychological insights from which to experience and analyse the problematical material brought to the group. Sometimes it will appear surprising to the protagonists that the director does not immediately take up the presented 'surface' problem but continues to explore with the protagonist features of the problem that may lie at a deeper and, perhaps, earlier level of experience. This is an example of a therapeutic approach that puts diagnosis and exploration high in the agenda of concern, the assumption being that once the correct diagnosis of the problem is discovered and revealed, then a means may be found of resolving it to the protagonist's satisfaction. An adjustment is then made. But here is another view of psychodrama, which is quite different. I quote from Kellermann (1992):

> In existential psychodrama there is no concept of health, normality or pathology and diagnosis is therefore irrelevant and unnecessary. Psychodrama is 'not therapy' in the medical sense of the word, but an emotional experience within the framework of an interpersonal encounter with spiritual values of its own . . . the goal is not to produce a cure but simply to become as spontaneous and creative as possible.

This seems to me to beg a number of very difficult issues. Human beings do wish to find a 'cure', no matter how that is defined, and for many people becoming more spontaneous and creative in the 'here and now' is the essence of the cure for them, because it is simply the absence of these qualities in their ongoing relationships that have brought them to the therapy group in the first place. They felt stuck. Hence my belief in the view of the director's part as an 'interpreting psychologist' in the process of the psychodrama. Readers may associate this with the well-known notion of the psychoanalyst making interpretations of the client's use of language or images. Indeed there is a connection. As clients we may not see the wood for the trees. Sometimes the therapist has to make an interpretation that draws our attention to our inability to see or hear an obvious emotional prompt. But just as an incompetent, insensitive psychoanalyst may 'tell' the client the meaning of a phrase or image without the active participation of the client, so the psychodramatist might push a client into a piece of action out of impatience with the client's stubborn refusal to 'see the obvious'. In my own practice, in whatever mode I am working, I have given an invitation to my client to consider other meanings with the words 'perhaps' or 'maybe'. Then if the 'interpretation' is acceptable I asked the client to consider and evaluate the suggestion. And so the stuckness may be relieved. It must always be remembered that an interpretation is an inspired piece of guesswork on the part of the therapist. It is a product of cognitive insight and imagination, based on what the therapist 'knows' about her client. It cannot be known to be 'true' or 'right' until the client tests it.

Kellermann rather arbitrarily attributes the process of looking for a cure to a behavioural existential approach. I am not sure what he means by behavioural and whether he includes psychoanalytic psychotherapy within that definition but it is certain that, in our own time, 'behavioural' tends to mean that which is strictly in the realm of the rational conscious ordering of behavioural management. Thus patients following a behavioural programme of therapy are educated into new behavioural habits, which can be detected as residing in the conscious mind. The problem arises when the difficulty being addressed is not amenable to rational adjustment. This is where non-behavioural interventions are required. Psychodrama can be very effective in this area, in as much as it often opens up and reveals emotional states that have been repressed and, in this state of repression, have effected an unconscious influence on the life of the person concerned. This was evident in the example quoted above, where repression had played a significant part in the complex of the mental state with its behavioural consequences. In our present state of knowledge the psychodrama director needs to acknowledge the influence of the unconscious within the mental life of us all, taking it into account as he prepares a client for performance.

There is no doubt that Moreno undermined the influence of psychoanalysis in his advocacy of psychodrama as a therapy. He insists on 'action' and 'motor events' in an article specifically addressing the attributes of therapy within psychodrama, as if the phenomenon of humans 'in action', physically or verbally and emotionally, is uninfluenced by the unconscious mind. It is as if Freud had never written *The Psychopathology of Everyday Life* or proposed the idea of patients 'acting out' old remembered pathological behaviour, as a defence against anxiety and the need for change. Most of us are aware of impulsive and non-rational behaviour that we have experienced when the unconscious has momentarily taken over control from the rational conscious mind. Sometimes we call it falling in love; sometimes we are merely drunk, either with alcohol, other drugs, or merely excitement.

Kellermann (1992) has given a comprehensive account of this early position, which Moreno took up, and readers who wish to pursue the topic may turn to his book for its quality of clear exposition in an area of confusion. I would only stress that as we proceed through this century we need to recognize that the psychological climate in the UK is very different from that which existed in the US many years ago. What emerges is the necessity for the psychodrama director to have achieved a position of relative theoretical sophistication in working through the method and current theories of psychodrama, some of which are complementary and others of which are in potential conflict.

The process of the director

In action this is based on her understanding and skill in working with the client's material as she moves into the psychodrama. We may delineate the process as a series of tasks.

- The task is to relate to the client in a manner that encourages and clarifies the client's concern, whilst at the same time remaining aware of the perceptual process within herself. Most of us will hear what we want to hear and see what we want to see!
- Alongside this developing working alliance comes a need to form an emotional resonance to the client whereby the director is able to move into close emotional harmony with the client whilst at the same time retaining the ability to keep a thinking therapeutic distance. Throughout these processes there remains a requirement to communicate clearly and openly with the client. The client is not present to be hoodwinked or treated as anything less than an equal partner. This may well mean that the director has to address barely revealed painful communications in such a way as to open them up to honest scrutiny. The client may be free to correct or challenge the communication of the director – this challenge being met with respectful attention by the director. A director may well make an observation that seriously misinterprets, or simply gets wrong the actual nature of a relationship the

protagonist is presenting. I can remember on one occasion mistaking a female aunt as coming from the mother's side of the family. She didn't. She came from the father's family; she was his sister. Very important. The protagonist eventually put me right. If she hadn't it would have been the job of an auxiliary therapist to do so.
- The director becomes an artistic director as the process matures. The director, working in close co-operation with the protagonist, moves him into the stage action place and they then set about furnishing the space with the minimum number of props and pieces of furniture to illustrate the chosen scene. At this point it is important that the *protagonist* chooses the props and furniture and physically sets out the arrangement to his own satisfaction. All this is observed by the director and the group and is considered therapeutic material of the first order. It may be commented upon, interpreted and symbolized as the situation suggests. As the action moves from warm up to action the director brings into place a whole armoury of techniques to enable the protagonist to explore and play with a series of emotional and imaginative propositions. The director is using her intuitive skills and practical knowledge of the theatre and the resources of psychodramatic skills that have been learned in her training. Competencies cannot be learned from a book such as this. The training group is the classroom of experience.
- The director needs to remember, however, the force of her interventions, whatever character they may take. The intervention may be verbal, using a double or speaking directly to the protagonist, or it might be non verbal. For example, simply mirroring the gestures, body position and body mood of the protagonist, either by using an auxiliary ego, or the self, to show the protagonist a conflict, or contradiction, between word and appearance, is a very powerful intervention.
- The director emerges clearly as the psychotherapist who, understanding the protagonist's messages of confusion, may offer clarity and understanding to the scene. One of the most difficult aspects of the director's therapeutic role is that of the person who challenges or addresses defensive behaviour on the part of the protagonist. This may arise out of contradictions and words of denial in the action of the drama, or it might come to notice by slips of the tongue or mistakes made by the protagonist in performance. For the psychodramatist, coming from an analytical background, this situation is not an unfamiliar one and is not a matter of conflict. For psychodramatists of other therapeutic training, coming to work in the field of psychodrama, this can be contentious. *Person-centred* psychotherapists for example, often find the concept of resistance and the issue of how such a manifestation is addressed, a difficult one to resolve. Traditional

followers of Moreno will talk about following and working with the resistance (Willis, 1991). The problem, here, is that too often it is not at all clear how this is to be achieved. Resistances can prove to be dogged, inflexible and intractable, a source of much frustration for the psychodrama director who rejects confrontation with the protagonist.

In another context Marcia Karp, the principal advocate and trainer in psychodrama in the UK, has a neat anecdote that she quotes (Holmes and Karp, 1991). It illustrates a confident and experienced psychodramatist, confronting a would-be protagonist in a very direct way. She tells her that merely to attend a number of unrelated sessions over a period of time is a waste of her time; she should come to the psychodrama centre and do a serious block of work. Implicitly Karp is recognizing the way in which a protagonist uses a way of 'coming and going' to the group as a way of avoiding work in depth.

Up to this point I have been addressing the place of the director as the artistic director and therapeutic stage manager, but the director's role is dynamic and the latter stages of the psychodrama, before it closes, call on the director to become a skilful group facilitator and analyst, requiring yet more attributes and performances.

The director is a *boundary keeper* and facilitates the closure of the psychodrama, ensuring a good end. The tracking process, described earlier, is an essential feature of this responsibility. The director will remember the starting point of the drama and where the individual members of the group placed themselves, emotionally, at its inception.

Now the protagonist is back in the group space. Literally sitting alongside his colleagues, the material of the psychodrama begins to emerge as a matter of group concern. We all know that, when an individual describes a problem, we all resonate to it in one degree or another. At this stage it is the job of the director to encourage the group to acknowledge their shared concern, even to identify, too, those in the group who were deeply involved in the action and to offer them recognition and space for expression. Perhaps the most important rule to be observed is to respect the need for the protagonist to close the drama. Therefore the group members use the sharing time not to interpret and extend the protagonist's material but, rather, to reflect on their own experience of the psychodrama. This is especially true of the experience of the auxiliary figures who have often played very demanding roles. In Chapter 2 I described the feeling of an auxiliary who had been cast as a dominating, macho figure, who accepted the role and then came to reflect upon it ruefully. This activity reassures the protagonist that the group has been in the process with her. This helps to resolve any feelings of isolation or pathology that the protagonist may be left with. I have already mentioned that this period is a time of acute observation for the director who will quickly become aware of key issues for individual members, which may call for work in succeeding sessions.

Sharing may well be the time when transference feelings are expressed directly towards the director. Especially if the psychodrama has worked upon intense parental, sibling and son/daughter themes. These feelings need careful handling. Firstly the genuineness of the feeling must not be denied or analysed in a manner that infantilizes or demeans the members of the group in any derogatory way. As to the repercussions within the director, Gillie Ruscombe King (Holmes and Karp, 1991) draws attention to the power of transference and to the need of the psychodramatist to keep an *enabling distance* from the feelings that may arise in herself, when developing a relationship with the client. I use the term enabling to indicate that the director needs to examine any feeling in herself that may or may not be attributed to transference affects. Distance here does not mean aloofness, avoidance or rejection, but rather the position a psychotherapist has to take up in order to effectively scrutinize her own inner world of feelings.

In this chapter I have outlined the basic position of the psychodramatist. Clearly therapists come to psychodrama from a number of different therapeutic perspectives. These perspectives, underpinned by a theoretical position and clinical practice, need to be incorporated into the practice of psychodrama, often amended to allow a creative experience for the director and her protagonist. Readers from these different psychotherapeutic positions will have to negotiate their own position and I hope this chapter, dealing as it does with the general position of the director, proves to be assistance without being narrowly prescriptive.

Chapter 8

Interlude

I close this account of the director's role with a summary of the basic techniques and instruments that are available to the practice of psychodrama within almost any approach.

The empty/auxiliary chair

This is perhaps the most flexible and easiest of techniques that the director may place at the disposal of the protagonist. Simply put, it means that an empty chair can be introduced into the acting area and held to represent a significant figure in the protagonist's life. It may be occupied by an auxiliary player to represent the figure or left empty. The chair can be used to represent parts of the protagonist's personality or life history – for example 'this chair represents me as I was ten years ago' or 'this chair represents my desire to please and my fear of disapproval!'

I recall, once, in my own experience as a protagonist, placing chairs in a circle to represent every 10-year anniversary in my life. I got as far as the sixth chair and then the notion of approaching death began to seep into my consciousness. It was a salutary experience. Now I would have to place a seventh chair in the circle!

The chair can be used in any way the imagination suggests. Sometimes it is a symbolic object, representing a thing of great value or a place of significance and so on. The only absolute rule is that, as the drama concludes, the protagonist de-roles the chair, strips away the symbolism and returns it to its humble significance as a chair.

Role reversal

This is at the very heart of Moreno's method. It is in essence a very simple but profound technique. Anyone can do it. The person chosen simply chooses a significant figure from her life and changes places with that figure. So A becomes B and B becomes A. I remember, in my early days, being impressed and amused at an anecdote that reported Moreno as changing places with a small boy, aged about eight years. The boy stood on a table and Moreno sat on the floor and a dialogue took place. I cannot vouch for the literal truth of this anecdote, and it may seem apocryphal, but the image is powerful and provides both insight into the technique and the nature of Moreno and his relationships with children.

In a psychodrama the protagonist simply briefs the person who is playing the reversed role. At first sight this seems amazingly complex, but I think this small extract from a drama will illustrate the method:

Scene 32

A clinical psychodrama group in a therapeutic community. Joan has opted to have a talk with her mother. At this point she has decided on duologue with an occupied chair. An auxiliary member of the group, Hilary, is to sit in the chair representing Joan's mother. But first she needs to be briefed. At this juncture Joan could warm up the person playing her mother by standing behind her and doubling. That is simply speaking in her mother's voice. I would often suggest the opening for the protagonist by cueing her to start by simply saying: 'my name is . . . I am . . . years old . . . I am . . . mother/sister/wife/girlfriend of and so on. The important feature being that the protagonist is speaking in the first person all the time. However, Joan, being a very experienced patient, chooses a modified variation of this approach, very effectively as it works out.

Joan (speaking from mother's chair; the auxiliary, Hilary, is now in Joan's chair): 'What on earth am I doing here at my age? Sixty-two last birthday! I should have thought Joan could well manage without me by now. After all she is not a child. And look at me, my hair is a mess and I certainly wouldn't have worn these old trousers if I had known I was coming. I would have worn my black skirt and boots with my leather jacket. Well never mind, can't do anything about it. What do you want, Joan? I can't stay long. Load of shopping to do and your father's lunch to get. He doesn't like to be late so what am I here for? Well I certainly didn't expect to find myself here at all, so let's get on with it.'

At this point the actors change place and Joan is now back at her chair and Hilary, playing mother, is in mother's chair. Hilary is fussing with her hair and looking around with a distrustful look on her face. Joan looks composed and speaks.

Joan: 'You don't need to do anything mother, or say owt for that matter. Just sit still, if you can, and listen [she pauses] if that's possible.'

Hilary (as mother, getting into the role): 'No need to be sarky, I told you Joan, I got your dad's dinner to get, I can't stay long.'

She moves as if to get up.

Joan: 'Sit still mum, just sit still please, I've got something to say, and I want you to hear it.'

Hilary sighs and slumps back into her chair in a posture of indifferent resignation. The role players reverse roles again and 'mother', now played by Joan, continues to pour out sceptical remarks about the intended conversation.

And so the drama continues. It will stay as a duologue, with interventions from the members of the group who will double as they see the relationship unfold. The director will, from time to time, check out the validity of the words and actions, perhaps highlighting body postures though mirroring techniques. Reverse role-playing is an invaluable technique for getting into someone else's position – getting into their shoes, as it were.

Often there is no need for an auxiliary to assist. John, a member of Joan's psychodrama group, for example, in a reverse role scene, simply took on his father's role and in that persona described how the father felt about John the son. The outcome was material that was rich and abundant. There was no need for any warm up or preparation. John could enter straight into the father's role without difficulty. In effect it was a soliloquy – which I describe in the next paragraph.

Soliloquy

Joan might have chosen to use the method of soliloquy to express her confused thoughts and feelings about her mother. Most of us are accustomed to the theatrical version of this technique. In Shakespeare, as the audience, we are not at all surprised if the character steps momentarily out of the action and addresses us directly to expose a predicament or a train of thought. It is a convention that is well understood and accepted. Even in modern plays and productions on television, occasionally, the producer introduces a moment when the actor speaks directly in this way. Brecht made good use of this technique. It is often a moment of theatrical intimacy when the audience and performer come close together.

In the circumstance of Joan's meeting with her mother, Joan might well have hesitated at the door to the room, wherein her mother sat waiting for her. Standing on the threshold she might well have indulged in a soliloquy in which she would expose, examine and explain, as well as she could, her relationship with her mother and her reasons for bringing her to the psychodrama. Readers will know how any one of us might use a soliloquy to rehearse for a meeting. Especially if it is a meeting we approach with nervous anticipation. Of course this voicing of our concerns usually goes on inside our heads. But sometimes, sitting at the traffic lights, we can observe other people, in their cars, talking away to themselves and it is quite reasonable to assume they might be rehearsing a coming encounter. Note that Joan could have shown us her mother via a mother's soliloquy. This could easily be done before any meeting of the two characters.

Doubling

This is a key technique in psychodrama. It's a most versatile and creative approach by which group members are enabled to enter the world of the protagonist. It is a method by which the director can enter the action either directly or through the agency of the auxiliary therapists. It rests upon our ability to empathize and identify with the protagonist. It comes into play, too, when members of the group gain an insight into the drama being enacted and try out the insight through a double, which will be accepted or rejected by the protagonist. Blatner (1973) thinks the topic so important that he devotes an entire chapter to discussing the technique. He describes the person who is doubling in the following simple terms:

> Consider this person, your double, your invisible self, your alter ego with whom you may talk at times, but who exists only within yourself. He may say things you may be feeling – things you would be hesitant to express. If his statement represents your true feelings, repeat that statement in your interaction . . . If what the double says is not an expression of your feelings, you are free to correct him, to say 'no'. This will negate what he says. If you, the protagonist, feel the double is unable to empathise with you, you may indicate this, and we (the director) will replace him.

Blatner puts this very clearly and very simply; his observations need to be followed in the work of psychodrama. There is no restriction on who may double for the protagonist or for any other character in the drama but there is a requirement on the part of the director to ensure the statement 'doubled' is heard clearly, then accepted and repeated, clearly, by whoever the double is attached to; or rejected, its rejection being made clear. This business of clarification is very important and the director has to be close enough to the action to participate and anticipate where it is leading, whilst at the same time watching and hearing all the participants in the drama. This is the function of tracking, which has already been discussed.

Doubling is essentially concerned with expressing feelings. The greater part of interventions of this kind come from the members of the group, but if none is forthcoming then the director may offer a double, more often than not, in my own practice, by using a co-therapist auxiliary. The following scene illustrates this in action.

Scene 33

A clinical psychodrama group in a therapeutic community. Mary is offering a psychodrama where she shows her voyeuristic self. She likes to watch events, preferably secretly. Her divorced mother has recently taken a lover. She sometimes makes love with him in the sitting room of the family house in the evening when Mary is supposedly in her bedsitting room, on the next floor. Quite heavy 'petting' takes place and so far the couple have not practised sexual intercourse with each other. They do not know they are being secretly observed by Mary.

The sitting room door is not quite closed and Mary's mother is spread-eagled on the sofa her lover lying against her. He strokes her and they exchange passionate kisses. Mary, seen by the therapy group, but not seen by the lovers is watching in silence. The director invites her to describe what she sees and in a very controlled voice she begins:

Mary: 'Look at them they are kissing. Look at the way my mother's dress is riding up her legs. He is all over her. He should keep his hands to himself. She shouldn't let him.'

All this comes out in a very quiet voice, barely heard by the group, with very little emotion allowed in the voice. Suddenly one of the group members goes to double. The double is almost an exact repeat of Mary's words except now they are infused with feeling. The double ends with the woman group member bringing her voice to a crescendo, virtually screaming.

Double: 'It's disgusting, absolutely disgusting; she knows I'm in the house. Fancy snogging here in our own living room with this terrible man. It's disgusting. No wonder Daddy left.'

As the double ends Mary is now in tears, her face is red and blotched with emotion. The woman group member is hot and looking worried, she goes to leave the scene but I intervene.

Director: 'No, stay where you are. Let Mary recover herself and tell us what she is feeling and thinking about your powerful double.'

Gradually Mary becomes calm and reflective. When I am satisfied she is stable I ask her to repeat the double, if it genuinely reflects her true feelings. With difficulty she accepts the double and tries to speak again with the force of the double. But it is difficult and her version does not quite reach the level of the double. Nevertheless progress has been made. In this instance the double addressed the repressed emotions. But another double may have approached the situation more obliquely. Let us imagine the following.

Double: 'Just listen to my voice, I sound so quiet and sensible, no sign of what is going on inside.'

Or:

'Mother would be horrified if she knew what I am doing, but I don't care. She is showing herself up. Just look at what she is doing!'

In both of these instances the protagonist would have been controlling the situation, hiding behind her voyeurism. In reality she herself had no sexual life, had no boy friend and had not had one since leaving school. Her neurosis had steadily developed with the father leaving home and now Mary, herself, was very reluctant to leave the family home even for simple shopping needs. She had been diagnosed as agoraphobic. Fear of going out into the world outside. In reality she was frightened of leaving the house 'in case'. It was not so much the issue of going into a strange world that frightened her as leaving the worrying and conflictual world of home where anything might happen in her absence. Where she would, by going out, lose control.

Doubling has many applications and, for example, a double may take the form of an auxiliary playing the part of an aspect of the protagonist. For instance, a client may have a public personality of conformity and politeness and a repressed aspect that is non-conforming and anything but polite. The director may well set up a dialogue or social situation where these aspects address each other. Sometime more than one double may be present, representing other aspects of the person. In the case of Mary it would have been useful to have a woman play her sexual being and the frustration that she felt, at the way in which sexual experience was only allowed in this voyeuristic, displaced way. The possibilities for the use of doubles is almost endless but the rule remains the same, the 'truth' of the double must be checked out with the person on the receiving end of the double. This is especially true when the double is sarcastic or satirical. Although both of these responses at the right moment may be valid if applied with understanding and sensitivity.

Note the difficulty in this scene, for the auxiliaries playing mother and lover. Practised professional actors can create a sexual love scene on the stage without too much difficulty and audiences accept this as a stage convention and do not regard it as obscene or perverted. But for clients in a psychodrama group it is a very different matter. My way of dealing with it is to ask the players to symbolize the action in a sculpture and then freeze it for the benefit of the scene. Hence in the scene described the woman auxiliary, playing the lustful mother, would certainly have 'spreadeagled' herself on the settee. And her dress could have been allowed to ride up her leg sufficiently to indicate her sexual desire and pleasure, but only to the extent that she, as an auxiliary, felt comfortable. The man auxiliary, playing the lover would have done something similar. His clothing could have been disarranged a bit, tie taken off, shirt undone. And then he could be invited to lean over the woman auxiliary in a pose suggestive of lovemaking and at this point be told to freeze. This would be the moment that the protagonist, Mary, would start to make her comments. Throughout this preparation the director's job is to ensure the safety of the performers, the protagonist, and the group as a whole. Obviously it is of advantage if the director has experience as an actor or director in the performing arts as a background to her work in therapy. No doubt in the sharing much will come out about the sexuality of those concerned.

Sometimes, however, doubling has its own disadvantages. The most obvious problem with doubling is that the subject of the double may be at the receiving end of other people's projections, which will almost certainly be a distorted reality, belonging to the doubler, little concerned with the reality of the main subject.

The director has a special responsibility towards the protagonist in this respect. She should watch, too, the physical proximity of the doubling group member to the protagonist. The best position for the 'doubler' to take up, physically, is at an angle to the protagonist, so that her face may be seen without difficulty. It is quite normal for the 'doubler' to place a hand on the protagonist's shoulder. It is a useful cue to the protagonist that a double is about to occur. Sometimes a protagonist is so immersed in the drama that she fails to notice the movement towards her of a group member wanting to double. But again the director should watch all these gestures carefully to ensure the safety of the protagonist and her freedom to accept or reject a double message. The director would be well advised to ask the doubler to retain contact with the protagonist until the message is clearly heard, accepted and repeated, or refused.

Blatner suggests a number of warming-up techniques to train people in the art of doubling. One of my favourites is to ask people to get into pairs and then person A sets out to describe herself to the rest of the group whilst the 'doubler', person B, adds a comment, which is based on the feelings the first person may have about herself.

This is a short example:

Miss A: Well, I am tall.

Miss B: Much too big.

Miss A: Rather brownish hair.

Miss B: It's mousy, shapeless and greasy.

Miss A: But I do have a nice smile.

Miss B: Which I *do* hope people will find attractive and like me.

And so on. When enough has been done the two women reverse roles. Remember, each time the director checks the comment out with the protagonist and then, if accepted, the comment is repeated.

The psychodramatic interview

The literature does not discuss the question of the director's interview with the protagonist very frequently, yet I consider it one of the most important pieces of action in an emerging psychodrama. My view is that the psychodrama interview starts as the protagonist emerges from the group. From this opening exchange in the circumference of the group the director opens up the working space and, accompanied by the protagonist, moves from sitting in the group's circumference to the dramatic space where action can take place. Once the director and protagonist are in this space then an interview can take place at a more intensive, therapeutic level. An interview is just what is implied by the term, in its everyday use. The director is there to explore with the protagonist the main features of the problem, dilemma or life situation that the protagonist wished to work with in the psychodrama. The other part of the interview, working at quite another level, is the director's need to understand, *in a psychotherapeutic way* the true nature of the conversation and to attempt to formulate an approach to the psychodrama. Formulation is a major part of any psychotherapeutic interview.

When I work as an analytic psychotherapist the first two or three interviews with my client are used, in part, to attempt a formulation, a guide to the future of therapy, and a guide to therapeutic aims and emphasis within the therapeutic alliance. Virtually all psychoanalytic trainees are subject to this approach and discipline. The task for the psychodramatist is much the same. The perception of 'what is wrong' by the director may not be the same as that of the protagonist. The material given to the director, in the interview, might suggest a different approach to the way the 'problem' is being described by the protagonist, with a consequent different approach implied, to working in the drama. It is a complex matter and the psychodramatist will have to work this out with the protagonist before any committed drama takes place. On the other hand, it also has to be recognized that a drama can change course and frequently does so when the material begins to emerge in action and reaction through the process of exposure and spontaneous dramatization. It is this flexibility and improvisatory, spontaneous activity that gives psychodrama its special quality. It should also be remembered that the whole group hears this interview, which acts an important briefing for those who may find themselves, at a later stage, playing a role or doubling.

Mirroring

This a relatively simple technique similar to sculpting. All of us, at some time, have caught a glimpse of ourselves in a mirror, in a public situation, and have not quite recognized the self, mirrored, that we see. Auxiliary therapists are often used to let the protagonist 'see' a reflection of their sometimes unconscious physical gestures, mannerisms, postures that all carry a message. One of the most obvious examples that comes to mind is of a client who habitually put his hand in front of his mouth, virtually every time he spoke in the psychodrama. Imagine his discomfiture when he realized that no less than three auxiliary actors were walking around the scene with their hands over their mouths.

On another occasion an auxiliary might sit beside a protagonist and mirror the gestures the protagonist is using, in the scene being enacted.

Sculpting

Sculpting is a very close relative to mirroring but it has a function of its own. The first and probably primary difference is that a sculpt is a static representation of a place, a situation, a figure, a meaning, or, most important, a feeling.

A single member of the group can enact a sculpt if required to do so, but it is more likely that a part of the membership of the group will get together to devise a sculpt. On occasions the whole group may construct a sculpt and this is particularly useful when the members want to say something about the dynamics of their group and the director. A simple example of this is when the director stands or sits in the centre of the group and invites members to place themselves in relation to him using not only space as a measurement of closeness and distance but taking up a pose to reflect their feelings about their relationship with the director. The possibilities of the sculpt are pretty well endless and often it can be used by the director, when meeting a group for the first time to establish, very quickly, the feeling that are emerging from the group towards its very being and its tasks as a therapy group.

Some time ago I was invited to visit a group analysis training group to talk to them about psychodrama and the use of action techniques in group therapy. I decided to use the experience of the group itself to warm us up to the possibilities of action techniques. I simply asked them to place an object in the middle of the room to symbolize the nature of their training course and then to place themselves physically in relation to the object, using distance, posture, and gesture as a symbolization of their feelings towards the training. Attending the group that night was a significant figure from the training therapist. He took the opportunity to take part in the exercise. When it was concluded the group came together again and discussed what they had seen and compared what individuals had assumed about one another before the exercise with what they had seen in the sculpt. There was an animated discussion and the strong feeling was expressed towards the group analytic therapist, who had clearly shown himself to be moving steadily away from the training course, placing himself at some distance from the symbolizing object and placing his body in the position of withdrawal. This, no doubt, would have provided rich material for subsequent meetings of the group.

Chapter 9

The protagonist

'And one man in his time
plays many parts,
His acts being seven ages.'

Shakespeare. *As You Like It.* Act 2, Scene 7.

The leading role

In this chapter I shall be examining the role of the protagonist in close-up. Some of the material will be theoretical, examining the phenomenon of role play and the manner in which it has come to a central position in psychodrama, but most of this chapter will be given over to experiential material drawn from my own experience as a protagonist and from that of clients who have worked with me in that form, in the National Health Service and private groups, when I have been in the role of director or co-director.

Role play has a long and interesting history. It has been a phenomenon of interest to sociologists, social psychologists, historians and psychotherapists throughout the twentieth century. The *Pocket Oxford English Dictionary* defines 'role' as an 'actor's part', a 'person on whom others model themselves' and 'acting of characters or situations as an aid in therapy, language teaching, etc.' This implies that much of role play is the 'as if' feature that comes across a good deal in psychodrama, where the protagonist and other players take on the position of someone else 'as if' they were that person, with interesting results. It is often an amazingly quick way of seeing a different point of view. In this instance there is a consciousness of 'playing a part' like an actor. We know, too, that people can play a role entirely unconsciously, without thinking about it, or copying someone else and psychodrama allows for both forms of role play. The latter has a more spontaneous quality than the former and therefore is nearer to the 'play' of children. However, children too are capable of copying the performances of those about them in their environment in quite a conscious way.

Quite what my dictionary intends by 'etc.' I am not sure. The dictionary ignores the way in which role play came to be a socially defined concept, for example accepting the role of *commander* of the troops in battle; a *director* of a business company, a *trade union leader* and so on. These are prescribed roles with particular social expectations. To some extent the 'script' is provided and a range of behaviour is expected of the player, that fits into the expectations. What lies behind this statement is the notion that being commander of troops has certain general, but specific requirements, which are applicable to any individual who takes on the position. It would be possible to write a 'job description' of the position as commander of troops for anyone wishing to take on that task. It would then be a guide to behaviour for anyone taking the post. Role, in this sense, is frequently associated with work and tasks. People talk about having a role to play in some vocational project. It is a highly functional concept. In most respects, as these roles are designated, we do not have to invent them when we are cast in such a role – we know more or less what is expected. We all play many roles during our lifetime. We take on a role as a task and perform it to satisfy an expectation of a social audience (Kellermann, 1992).

As far as therapy is concerned, we recognize the value of the word 'role' in thinking about other socially defined activity. We have a concept of *mothering* and *fathering*, which is general – it goes beyond any particular interpretation and is usually culturally bound. In other words, in Britain we hold certain ideas about being a mother or father, which are shared throughout the community, interpreted by the class and ethnic background from which the ideas emerge. Many of Freud's ideas about mothering and fathering were tightly culturally bound by his background of Jewish identity, by being professional, and middle class in aspiration and manner, by living in Vienna at a particular moment of time and by being raised primarily within a Victorian value system. Clearly, to be a mother or father in a remote part of Uzbekistan or Africa would have certain characteristics that would be unique to the practices and culture of the community in which the role was being enacted. On the other hand we would not be surprised to see certain aspects of the role that were held in common with our own. The universality of some values and role performances seems to be expected by us all from whatever background we come from.

Schutzenberger (1975) writes in some detail about role. She writes 'each person acts "normally" without realising they are in role . . . Goffmann sees people as continuous actors, co-acting at the same time in everyday life a number of roles . . . [they] prepare unconsciously to perform in public – the schoolroom, living room with guests, or entering a good restaurant.'

Schutzenberger suggests that we learn our roles from the principal figures of influence in our life and our range and flexibility in performance will rest to some extent on the quality of that learning. As a psychoanalytic therapist I would include, within that concept, the unconscious emotional 'learning' that occurs in the very early formative period of our lives, our childhood, it resonates upon our personality and emotional interpersonal relationships for the rest of our lives. Schutzenberger argues that the structure of these role performances is very complex, informed and influenced as they are by interaction from those around us, from other performers, who in turn are influenced by us and our special way of performing. It is obvious that the possibilities are endless and that flexibility and new learning is essential if human beings are going to remain emotionally healthy throughout their lives.

This was Moreno's position and his book *Who Shall Survive?* (1934) is an elaboration of these ideas together with the idea that our survival depends upon our ability to confront life in the 'here and now', not repeating and depending upon the practice of the past, especially where it is inappropriate. Kellermann (1992), in dealing with the suggestion that performing 'as if" roles somehow lacks genuineness and encourages a 'false self', attributes the following to Janov (1970): 'psychodrama does not employ role playing and "as if" to develop a false self . . . rather (it's) a way to expand the various parts of self through activity.' The 'activity' is playing the role of other significant others in the life of the performer, or trying out a new life position or attitude as a response within the psychodramatic performance. Role reversal is the most obvious example of how this taking on another point of view or attitude may be explored by a protagonist to her benefit. Simply speaking through your mother's voice and experience can be a revelation. Most performers find that when they step into such a position they find that earlier prejudicial blocks to their understanding are, in that moment, removed.

Schutzenberger's assertion that we are largely unconscious of the roles that we are preparing, rehearsing and playing is central to the suggestion, in this book, that psychoanalytic theory may inform the practice of psychodrama, to the advantage of the practitioner, if she should so desire to enter that world. However, some psychodramatists have found it difficult to acknowledge this view, being mindful of Moreno's known antagonism to psychoanalysis and to its founder, Freud. As an aside I sometimes imagine Moreno and Freud in a role-reversal situation. We can put aside old antagonisms and look more clearly at the proposition that the unconscious influences not only the protagonist in the playing of a role but also the director (after all, that is role too) and the group. Similarly psychoanalysts in the UK have been slow to recognize the importance of psychodrama. Few have any skill in that direction, although, as stated earlier, Foulkes, an early founder of group analysis here in the UK, did recognize its importance. Rarely do textbooks on psychoanalysis consider the significance of the notion of role, or discuss role theory from a psychoanalytic point of view. Certainly, Melanie Klein showed no interest in the formation of role relationships, despite the fact that she was heavily influential in the UK thinking about the formation of the human personality. Her concerns came to be discussed at the British School of Psychoanalysis in the post-war period and many psychoanalysts framed their concepts around her theoretical propositions. Object relations theory places a heavy emphasis upon the search for relationship that all human beings pursue, but even such a distinguished 'object relations' theorist as Winnicott (1971), whilst recognizing the intrapsychic force of imaginative play in the child's formulation of its relationship with the outside world, tends to neglect the social psychological implication of this phenomenon in considering how a child learns.

Winnicott seems more interested in the inner dialogue of the child, its intrapsychic formulations in its relationship with its mother, rather than the social interrelationships that must spring up from the child's presence in a social world. I am reminded of very recently waiting at the doctor's surgery, where I had a very spirited non-word communication with baby of about 13 months. Sitting upon her mother's lap she found me an object of much amusement, as I did her! She was behaving socially in the 'role' of a baby, albeit unconsciously. I played the approving 'grandfather'. The child's mother found me to be an unthreatening presence as I played out this essentially benign role.

However, if we look abroad in Europe we find other countries where psychodrama has been successfully incorporated into the clinical culture. A good example is Hungary, where a number of distinguished psychologists and psychotherapists acknowledge and use the special qualities of clinical psychodrama in their practice and teaching. The mentor for these psychotherapists is Merei (1994), whose influence in Hungary can hardly be overstated. It might be argued, too, that psychodrama came to Hungary and received a sympathetic welcome following on the heels of the work of Sandor Ferenci, a colleague and contemporary of Freud, who challenged the notion of the therapist being a mirror-like creature in the eyes of the client, in favour of the therapist being a more active and caring figure of influence. This provoked a very spirited response from Freud. However, it is echoed in psychodrama by the role and place of the director in the protagonist's performance. This is not to suggest for a moment that the director is a sugary or sentimental figure – on the contrary, the director frequently introduces challenge and reality into a performance where conflict or contradiction is being avoided. It is a robust position.

Scene 34

Takes place in a training group. William is in full flood, addressing a sterile relationship that he has had with a young woman, Julie, for many years. He is married and this has been an 'extra marital' relationship, characterized by a lack of sexual contact and an obsessive degree of secrecy between William and his 'girlfriend' Julie. The relationship is heavily influenced by fantasy, from which William finds it very difficult to detach himself.

Director: 'William I suggest you reverse role with Julie for a moment and let's hear her account of the relationship with you, especially the fact that you apparently cannot be sexual with her.'

William: 'Well, I don't really want to be in bed with her. She is quite delightful as a person. I get a lot from her. I touch her in the car. I often drive with my hand on her leg and she will squeeze my hand, so we do have physical contact.'

Director: 'Are you saying you don't want to reverse role with her?'

William: 'Not exactly. But I don't see the point. I know what she thinks about me. She loves me I know that.'

The director beckons to his co-therapist and there is a low keyed, short conversation. The co-therapist moves behind William.

Co-therapist (doubling for William): 'I don't want to talk with her voice. She may well be seen by others as castrating me. I like things as they are. I don't feel threatened by her. Besides I might feel guilty. I probably shall. Joan, my wife knows nothing about this affair. It's being going on for years. It's my secret and Julie's secret. Her boyfriend knows nothing about this situation.'

Director: 'Well, William, true or false? Or, perhaps partly both. You can clarify all this. Shall we proceed?'

Notice the ambiguity of the phrase 'Shall we proceed?' Who is the 'we'? 'Proceed . . . to where, with whom?'

Here we see the director, through the agency of his co-therapist, putting enormous pressure on a client, using material that has emerged in the warm up part of the psychodrama to advantage in dealing with the client's resistances. The relationship is active and demanding without being persecutory and the protagonist may respond as he wishes. This is an example of a situation where William, the protagonist, will certainly not see playing the part of Julie as unrealistic make believe, fanciful and unconvincing. He knows that if he steps into her shoes then he might find himself confronting uncomfortable and difficult emotional material. Their collusive secrecy may well be exposed for the neurotic alliance that it seems to portray. The director knows, through William's choice of material for the psychodrama, that at a deep level he wants to expose this relationship and find a new way of managing it or abandoning it.

On the matter of resistance Willis (1991), in an interesting chapter on group analysis and psychodrama, illustrates the position of the director in dealing with resistance:

> The conductor [director] has very much the role of 'agent provocateur' . . . who when necessary drives events forward . . . the conductor [director] neither appears as a blank screen, nor risks too much personal transparency, but has to be reckoned with alongside of other(s).

The term *conductor*, used by her here, is drawn from formal group analytic language and is the equivalent of the term 'director' in the context of psychodrama. She goes on 'the basic rule is ultimately not to collude with or follow the patient's defensive moves, but to challenge them.' She continues by quoting Molnos (1987). 'Relentless pressure brings the resistance more and more into the open "intensifying the patient's anxiety until the true feeling is reached".' So this is the situation the protagonist might have to face.

Of course, the procedure has to be followed at the discretion of the director and she estimates how appropriate the pressure may be in helping a client reach a deeper level of experience, which is tolerable, with consequent insight and emotional learning. This experience is sometimes described as a 'corrective emotional experience'. It is possible that the pressure, if arousing intensive anxiety, might prove entirely counterproductive, the client becoming incapable of any personal analysis or therapeutic action. Furthermore, such misjudgement and application by the director, might well contradict the concept of psychodrama as being an avenue of spontaneity and play which is at the heart of Moreno's ideas concerning the nature of a therapeutic experience. Willis (1991) insists upon these aspects of therapy in her chapter introducing group analytic psychodrama, and my own experience of working playfully attests to the importance of these ideas. The following scene illustrates a moment when a psychodrama group begins to work with great playful imagination. The play has an edge to it and constituted a learning experience for the protagonist.

Scene 35

A training group in St Petersburg meeting on a regular basis. The group is well established and trusting and is capable of quick, spontaneous action. Natasha has been doing a psychodrama that contains both her anger towards her mother, who apparently failed to provide enough outward affection and care for her children, and Natasha's own fear that she may be smothering her six-year-old with too much love and attention. She is a single parent, very intelligent and sensitive, and she is aware that she may be using the child to compensate for the loss of her lover. The group is listening to her intently. Natasha is sitting on a sofa as she speculates about her condition. Then, without any prompting, a women from the group goes to the sofa and sits closely beside her, putting her arm around her. Natasha smiles gratefully, and then another woman comes and sits on the other side and holds her. She is still pleased. As director, I am intrigued. I half guess at what is going on. Then another woman psychologist, the youngest in the group, small and pretty, walks across and climbs on to Natasha's knee, wrapping her arms around her neck. Another woman, Sonia, walks behind her, kneels down, and puts her arms around the back of Natasha's neck. Natasha can now barely speak and wriggles, from to time to release herself, but it is no good. Then Igor, a young strong man, a junior doctor, walks across and tries to pull the women apart. They resist firmly. Nothing is said. The action continues. I decide to let the struggle continue for a while. Then the co-therapist, who is also well aware of the significance of all this, speaks to me.

I call out 'FREEZE'. Everyone does as I command. The co-therapist goes over and doubles.

Co-therapist as Natasha: 'Ok. I've got the point, you can let me go.'

I speak to Natasha as the director: 'Well Natasha, do you agree?'

Natasha grins at me and weakly nods.

I speak again: 'You're quite sure? You don't have to, you know that.'

She smiles at me broadly now and addresses her captors: 'Yes I've got the message, you can let me go and let Igor in.'

This they proceed to do and Igor climbs on her lap smiling and touching her face with his hand. After a few minutes he leaves her with a smile and goes back to the group circle. She smiles to the group and I close the action.

A small cultural footnote is called for here. To my surprise, when I first went to work in the then Soviet Union, I found that the professionals I trained welcomed and worked easily with physical contact, rather in contrast with my 'British' experience.

We talked in the group about the spontaneity of the action and, although Natasha had been speculating about her controlling feminine love, the group felt she needed to feel the pressure of so much attention, even when it looked affectionate and attentive. She was failing to notice how she kept men at bay. This is an example of how the whole group can behave spontaneously in showing the protagonist their view of what she is saying. They acted out their scepticism. They did not believe that her intellectual appraisal of her problem was connected closely to her feelings. The youngest of them quite spontaneously and playfully became her daughter and Igor chose just the right moment to approach her, as available men might do. This scene also shows how much the protagonist has to cope with. The emotional and physical pressure on Natasha was considerable. As director I let her 'suffer' the experience in order that she could enter the situation feelingly. Her former role of motherhood and womanhood was challenged in a powerful but amusing way. The group watching as the scene took place at first began to giggle and then to laugh out loud once they had got the meaning of the action. The two other men in the group were urging Igor on and burst into applause when he finally sat on her lap and stroked her face.

This next scene, in contrast to the last, shows how the protagonist becomes very powerful in the direction of her own psychodrama, using the group in a systematic and meaningful way. The background to the scene was quite straightforward. It concerned a client who had grown up in a family with very powerful and successful parents who had established a family culture of high and distinctive achievement. The client concerned, now living a separate and independent life of modest professional achievement, as a primary school teacher, still felt the presence and judgements of her parents and siblings keenly. She wanted to explore this situation and take some action to reduce the perceived critical presence of her family in her own appraisal of herself.

Scene 36

A psychodrama training group of some standing, meeting weekly. Fatimah, of Asian origin, a member of the group, has decided to explore the family situation, described above, through the process of sculpting. She uses almost all the group members to help her. At first she calls them out one after the other and ascribes roles to them. At the same time she gives 'nutshell' descriptions of the status of the family member concerned and calls on the player to stand in a certain space in relation to herself, the distance and posture and positioning of the family member representing Fatimah's view of their existing emotional relationship. At the same time the brother, sister, mother or father recounts, out loud, the achievements of his or her professional position.

Readers will probably have recognized the approach as a form of family sculpting. It is a very quick and affecting way of portraying family dynamics and is often used in family therapy.

The sculpt proceeded. The family figures spontaneously grew louder and louder in their personal vocal statements as they struggled to be heard, one against the other. In the middle of the sculpted circle stood Fatimah. She looked around herself with a mixture of angry amusement and confusion. She spoke several times, but no one heard her, or if they did, they paid no attention to her.

As director I spoke to her loudly and affirmatively: 'Now Fatimah you will have to speak up if you are going to be heard. All this quiet, polite deferential behaviour is not going to get you anywhere. You don't have to be polite here.' Fatimah looked at me, questioningly. 'But they won't listen to me, they never have. They can't hear me because they are making so much noise. What a bloody noise! Listen to it!' Fatimah was quite fond of low-key swear words.

Director: 'Shall I stop them?'

Fatimah: 'Please do.'

Director: 'No. On second thoughts I think you had better shut them up. You put them there and you encouraged all this noise. So you shut them up.'

Fatimah: 'Damn, you are a devil, a proper devil, leaving it all to me. None of the men in our family ever backed me up, no not one of them.'

Director: 'So it's up to you.'

At this point Fatimah, muttered under her breath. It sounded like 'you sod' but I could not be sure. Then, standing up straight and tall, she shouted.

Fatimah: 'Shut up all of you, this instant.'

And they did. There was absolute silence. The next action by Fatimah was crucial. She took each family member in turn and repositioned them until the family group was now standing in a series of clusters, at a good distance. No longer a circle around her.

Fatimah: '*I couldn't hear myself think, couldn't hear myself speak. That's better. Now stay where you are. Oh, yes you can talk,* quietly *among yourselves, to yourselves, not to me. Yes, you are all bloody marvellous. And so am I. Do you hear? And so am I.* And so am I.'

In the sharing we all pointed out our own experiences of being a member of a family group and our role in the family, sometimes resisted, sometimes enjoyed, depending on the changing circumstance. We noted too, how playing the roles in such a narrow, stripped down way highlighted the need for achievement in our lives; a universal desire. We also recognized that if the achievement was to mean anything then it had to be recognized by others, so we had to make ourselves heard, like the family figures in the sculpt psychodrama. Members of the group linked these reflections with their class and cultural experiences in the host society of the UK. As director I shared the feeling of anger and exasperation that came towards me from the protagonist in the drama, which probably belonged to the men and women in the family.

Readers will have noted that my job as director in this piece of work was minimal. And it is often like this in psychodrama – once the characters have entered firmly into role and understand the process, the action proceeds with energy. The director's job is mainly to keep the interest of the protagonist firmly in mind and in focus, to monitor the process as it unfolds, so as to relate to the ongoing work and to foresee future work to come, both for the protagonist and other members of the group. On the other hand I noted Fatimah's bitter remarks about the men in the family and her *sotto voce* attack on me for being a 'sod' leaving her to go it alone in sorting out the struggle.

It has to be remembered that it takes some courage for protagonists to come forward and offer to perform. In the instances just quoted both the protagonists admitted to feeling very nervous when they offered to work as protagonist. They felt, too, at some risk, wondering what was to become of them. They spoke of their relief at the end of the psychodrama, not only for the quality and worth of the work performed but also because they felt supported by the director and the group. Fatimah 'forgot', in her pleasure, that she had felt me to be a 'sod'. Both protagonists felt they had not been made to feel foolish or overexposed by the experience.

It is a necessary condition of good creative work in psychodrama that the protagonist should feel that the therapeutic support of the director is unconditional. All protagonists have the right to expect this support – that is, not without challenge, but always unconditional. Kellermann (1992) refers to a problem that might arise where the psychodrama group is a training group and the director is faced with the issue of giving feedback to a trainee psychodrama director, which may well include comments that could be construed as critical. Here the training director is faced with two loyalties. Firstly she must give therapeutic attention to the protagonist, ensuring the safety of the protagonist, and ensuring that the wellbeing and therapeutic aims of the protagonist are safeguarded. Secondly, she has to be fully supportive to the trainee director working with the individual so that the learning process is respected and protected. Balancing these positions is not always easy and Kellermann refers to a situation where the protagonist wanted to protect the trainee director from any critical appraisal, fearing an attack. This is not necessarily a transference issue. Indeed it may be much nearer to what Moreno describes as the presence of 'tele'. An energetic and creative alliance has been constructed during the period of the psychodrama, between the protagonist and the trainee and this is the relationship that appears to be threatened by interventions from the training director. Furthermore, even positive critical appraisal may appear to threaten the value of the work done by the protagonist in such a situation. The presence and activity of a co-therapist in this situation can be invaluable, interpreting and opening up the nature of the potential conflict, which, in turn helps to resolve it.

Scene 37

A training group in an NHS clinic. The membership is entirely professional including several psychiatrists, two of whom are consultants. One of these consultants, Alec, has no 'gift' for psychodrama and finds it painful to 'double', play a 'role', or take on the part of protagonist, although he participates in the sharing process in quite a relaxed fashion. He has not so far, in the life of the group, acted as a trainee director.

The training director has a dilemma. It is customary for individuals in the group to choose one of the members to act as director when choosing to do a psychodrama. So far no one has asked Alec, the consultant, to play that part and he has never been chosen to be a co-therapist by a trainee director. To try to move the situation forward the training director decides to direct the next psychodrama herself and invites Alec to work as co-therapist. A member of the group, Edward, comes forward to be the protagonist and accepts the suggestion of the training director to direct his psychodrama. Edward, the protagonist, is a junior doctor, specializing in psychiatry. Now the training director invites Alec to come into the acting space and work as co-therapist.

Director: 'Alec will you help me? I would like you to be my co-therapist.'

Alec: 'Me?'

Director: 'Yes you, Alec. Is that OK, with you?'

Alec: 'Well, I don't know. Do you think I can?'

There is a tense silence in the group. Everyone, including the protagonist, is looking anxiously at Alec.

Mary (a member of the group): 'Why not? She wouldn't have asked you if she thought you couldn't cope. I'm sure Edward would be glad if you did.'

There is a pause.

Edward (hesitantly): 'Yeah, that's fine by me. Of course I don't mind. Go on Alec. It will be good for both of us.'

The Training Director has noticed the phrase 'good for both of us'.

Director: 'Yes I'm sure that it will. You are all in the same boat here. Learning together. Helping each other. You know how the song goes: "With a little help from our friends." Bless the Beatles.'

There is a noticeable drop in tension. The group grin and giggle a bit at the reference to the Beatles and one of them, Miriam, begins to sing the words softly, some others join in, tentatively smiling at Alec. The atmosphere is becoming playful and more relaxed.

Alec: 'OK, but if I get in the way then perhaps you will just gently help me out.'

Director: 'Sure. Thanks. Let's get started. Oh, and the auxiliary players will support you Alec, so don't panic.'

But the director is yet again struggling with the old agenda. What is Alec doing in this group? Why did he sign up to stay after the introductory sessions? Perhaps he is only capable of being a patient. The psychodramatic training scene doesn't really support this situation. Maybe he should just go off and be a patient for a few years and then think about training. But he is a consultant and it will be difficult to own the position of patient. He has not had psychoanalytic training so he is not used to the idea of becoming a well-informed patient. These are the thoughts and dilemmas pursued by the director as she moves into action. Although this scene relates specifically to a training group, it is not entirely unusual to find a group member occupying such an ambivalent position in a therapy group. Indeed a number of clients attend clinical psychodrama groups and resist taking on the role of protagonist. It is as if they wish for a psychodramatic experience by a process of osmosis. They seem to believe that simply being there is enough to bring about change. But of course it is not. Like any psychotherapy, psychodrama requires participants to work directly for themselves.

To summarize, the therapeutic work elements of psychodrama for the protagonist may be seen as follows:

- the gaining of insight from exposure to the dynamics of personal and social relationships;
- the experience of sharing problems and personal material with others;
- the opportunity to rehearse new or different responses to either old or new problematical situations;
- to experience and express cathartic feelings that have been denied or repressed and which have proved, in the denial or repression, to be destructive within personal or social relationships;
- to experience a learning opportunity where both the conscious and unconscious self are addressed, offering the client new perspectives on the nature of self and the way that self is experienced by others.

I have, of course, subsumed within these categories many other qualitative experiences that the protagonist might gain from psychodrama psychotherapy but these five main headings seem to contain the major elements of therapeutic work that is experienced and fulfilled by a protagonist who embraces the therapy with integrity and a will to work honestly to a resolution.

Chapter 10

Members working together

'There is a history in all men's lives. . .'

Shakespeare, *King Henry IV, Second Part*, Act 3, Scene 1

There is a strong concept of the idea of *work* in the culture of psychotherapy. In individual work it is often seen as a form of alliance between the therapist and the client, working towards a common end, which is to fulfil the therapeutic aims of the client. In group work, of whatever chararacter, the concept is more complicated because there is an implicit presence of levels of work. There is the work required from each individual member to achieve personal therapy and then there is the need for the group members to work to help each other accomplish these personal aims. Finally there is a need for the group to work together to become a good working group. Psychodrama is interestingly a way of working that embraces all these aims and devises methods to accomplish them. In this chapter we shall examine how this comes about.

It is possible to use psychodrama as an individual encounter between therapist and client (Casson, 1997) and I have had this experience myself. In an encounter with an individual client in analytical psychotherapy my client suddenly took on her mother's voice and manner, as experienced when the client was about 12 years old (Feasey, 1999). I suppose that, without psychodramatic training, I might have been disconcerted by this experience but as a psychodramatist I was familiar with the occurrence – it did not alarm me, nor did I regard it as a pathological reaction by my client. I certainly did not regard her as hysterical, in the abusive use of that term. On the contrary I picked up her cue and merely responded by saying, 'I imagine this is your mother speaking, this is her voice.' For a moment she *acted out* a memory. Here I am using the term 'acting out' as Freud first intended. An old memory is behaved. My client was in imagination and memory 12 years old, in the family orchard with her beloved father, when her mother's intrusive voice was heard, loud, clear and condemning.

The remembered child's voice parodied that of the mother. She remembered it and spoke it. We all of us from time to time recall and use the voices of authority from childhood. It is not unusual. The unusual element is to offer the memory to a listener – in this case me. Sometimes, in supervision, I have found it very useful to ask the therapist in supervision to reverse role with a difficult manager or an obstructive colleague or a resistant client, simply to clarify and hold up to examination otherwise very confused material.

There should be no preconceived ideas about what the techniques of psychodrama can and cannot do. With imagination, creativity and spontaneity the techniques may be applied in numerous situations, the only limitation being the possibilities in the director's or protagonist's mind.

However, in this chapter I wish to look more closely at the psychodrama group through the eyes of a group psychotherapist who has trained in both a psychodrama group and an analytic group. At first acquaintance the contrast between the groups would seem extreme. In the analytic group the conductor appears passive and unresponsive, only rarely making an observation or interpretation. To some extent this will depend upon the model of group conductor the therapist is following. For example, someone who is heavily influenced by Bion (1961) will probably adopt the most remote and detached of stances, whereas someone who is closer to the tradition of Foulkes (1975) will probably take up a closer more available position for the group members, without entering into any excessive self disclosure. Foulkes (1975) in his chapter 'Diagnostics' describes the relationship between therapist and client:

> A degree of liking and trust develops. Even if things become difficult there is a foundation of goodwill and mutual respect which will see us through. It is important that a 'good therapeutic relationship' is not simply an expression of 'positive transference'.

I regard this as a most important statement, close to Moreno and Rogers. Here he is getting close to Moreno's *tele*. Yalom (1975) advocates an even closer position relative to the group membership then these others. He writes:

> Underlying all considerations of technique there must be a consistent, positive relationship between therapist and patient. The basic posture of the therapist to his patient must be one of concern, acceptance, genuineness, empathy. Nothing, no technical consideration, takes precedence over this.

Notice his stress on the word 'nothing'. I think readers would agree that this view is as much a matter of philosophy as psychology. For my own part I resonate closer to him and Foulkes than Bion.

The psychodrama director, by contrast, seems very active. An intervening and controlling figure, quick to comment and to act. But this is essentially a superficial view. It does not alter the fact that the reality of conscious and unconscious dynamics of the group are observable and worked with in both group settings. The director of psychodrama group and group conductor in an analytic group is as much involved in the dynamics of the group as anyone else. The essential question is what notice is taken of the manifestation of the dynamics in its conscious and unconscious presence within a psychodrama group – and by whom? The short answer is that it is impossible for the director not to take notice of the conscious dynamics of a group, whatever language is attached to its manifestation. For example, in the choice of protagonist in the group setting it is obvious that the director will notice avoidance as well as competitive and demanding bids for attention from group members. How the director works with this is another matter. What is more debatable is to what extent the director will observe and recognize the meaning of the unconscious group life and use it to the benefit of the members of the group, both individually and collectively. This latter position is often not attempted by psychodrama directors of the humanistic school.

Davies (1988) writes interestingly about the interpretation of the unconscious and he discusses the role of the director. He maintains the view that the director does not make open interpretations but waits upon the group to tackle unconscious group issues through the medium of the work proposed by an individual member. For example, rivalry for the attention of the director might easily be examined, in its psychoanalytical meaning, through a personal psychodrama, where the problem of siblings in the family group is addressed. What he does not say, however, is what to do if the group remains stubbornly resistant to *recognizing* and *acknowledging* unconscious group issues as they break through into the conscious life of the group. It is in this situation that the director may need to make a pertinent observation, linking one state of here-and-now concern with the repressed elements of group experience, which emerge, sometimes in a distorted version, from time to time. Barbara Jean Quin (1991) firmly rejects any form of interpretation in the sharing process, especially where it is directed towards the protagonist. This is the classical psychodramatic position. However when the director shifts attention to the group as a whole then another situation occurs (Willis, 1991). My own practice was to allow time for observations on the nature and state of the group when the main sharing activity was completed. At this time, depending upon the particular circumstances, sometimes in a follow-up session, I would pass an enabling observation, which would help the members to discuss their collective life as a group if they wished to do so, and in their own way. This could lead to some collective drama work where we would look at our shared experience of one another. In the group analytic movement this would be regarded as an 'intervention', but I avoid the use of this term, which I regard as too strong in its implications concerning the strength and authority of the group leader and the danger of the leader literally *getting between* the group members through an 'intervention'. I have always been puzzled as to how this term has been introduced into group analysis, with its implications of *getting between*. Strange. I would pass an *observation* or *comment*, offering it to the group to be taken up or abandoned as the case may be. Sometimes the director has to be very patient! Sometimes, in a psychoanalytical mode, the director might make an enabling interpretation to help the group move forward.

As regards the question of the way in which the group observes the group conductor or psychodramatic director, any reader of this book who has experienced any form of group psychotherapy will know the intense interest there is within the group concerning the leader. In some respects the more withholding the leader is, the stronger is the fantasy present in the group as members try to interpret the leader's presence, often unsuccesfully and with a degree of frustrated irritation and anxiety.

The psychodrama group is a working psychotherapy group and this is true, too, of the training group, although its form is sometimes different, bearing in mind the role of the director, in the latter case, as a teacher/evaluator as well as therapist.

In the group the members have a therapeutic job to do. Each and every individual has to work for the benefit of the other individuals and for the group as a whole. Although the director has the primary task as therapist, she is helpless unless the group members actively support the psychodramatic and learning process. The problem of how to 'teach' in a psychodrama training group is quite a critical one. My own practice has been to allow some separation of experience so that the critique, which is required from the teacher in response to the trainee's work as a director, comes *after* the therapeutic sharing. The group then can play a part in the process of feedback to the trainee where technical matters will predominate. It is important that the director holds the group to this task and does not let the boundaries slip into therapeutic discussion.

Let us look at some group tasks.

Choice of protagonist

The group plays a most obvious and open role in choosing the person who is to be the protagonist. There are many forms of pursuing this end, but finally the group has to decide and agree to whoever is proposed. A mature group, confident in its relationships, will tackle the job with understanding and confidence. The director works actively in the process and will make influential contributions to the decision, this being especially true when the director is trying to encourage a reluctant potential protagonist to perform. The director may offer some warm-up exercises to help the group reach a decision.

Provision of resources

The group provides resources to the protagonist in the form of persons able and willing to play *auxiliary roles* in the emerging psychodrama. This is of critical importance. Although it is possible for a protagonist to work effectively with a small cast of figures to support her drama, the contribution of the whole group is vital to the therapeutic process. This means that not only do group members as individuals accept the challenge of playing representational roles in the psychodrama – they also take on the work of *spontaneous* doubling. In this way the issues presented by the protagonist are gradually and effectively analysed, illustrated and understood. I use the term analysed here quite deliberately as doubling is a very effective form of analytic commentary when properly used. Moreno (1953) described the group members as therapeutic agents and practice confirms this conclusion. The element of *spontaneity* is central to the therapeutic process of psychodrama. Moreno (1953) thought of it as a way of responding in a new way to an old situation.

Scene 38

A clinical psychodrama group in a therapeutic community. The group is well established and its members have been working together for two months. John is complaining endlessly in his psychodrama about the way his mother controls his life, her persistent interference and her demands for an account of his every move. The group member playing his mother is very capable and forceful and is clearly enjoying her role of dominance and control. In an aside to the audience John has pointed out her enjoyment and how sadistic it is. A member of the group rises from his seat and approaches John. As director I give a brief nod to the member, offering support for his double. Interestingly I cannot, at this stage, know what the double is going to be, but I am pretty sure it is going to open something up for the group.

Fred, the double, speaks: 'Oh what a lovely time I am having. This woman, my mother – what a woman! – will never let me go. These fights draw us ever closer together. I could leave home tomorrow. I've a decent job, money in the bank and a girlfriend. No one can say I'm "gay" no one. But I'm not leaving mother, no way, she's not going to throw me out.'

The double finishes. I ask Fred to stay close to John. It is important that after a double has been given the speaker stays in position until the words have been acknowledged, accepted or rejected by the protagonist.

Director: 'Well, this is what Fred says you may be thinking and feeling beneath all this bluster. Perhaps he is revealing your hidden, or even your unconscious thoughts and wishes. What do you think?'

Pause.

Director: 'Any chance that he might be right?'

Unnoticed to John, but not to me, another group member, Evelyn, has come out to double for mother.

Evelyn: 'Oh, I love a good fight with John. Listen, John, to what I am saying. You know it's true, we are old sparring partners. You are thirty years old, and if you ever leave, which God forbid, I don't know what I'll do. Your father is a right drip.'

The rest of the group are grinning and laughing – not loudly, but clear enough for every one to hear.

John (responding to my question, now well aware of the doubles) replies: 'I don't know. I suppose it's a bit like that. Dad is a drip. She treats him like dirt, he does nothing. At least I stand up for myself.'

Director: 'And your girl friend?'

John: 'She thinks I am as soft as shit. Excuse the language.'

Director: 'It's certainly a bit smelly, isn't it. A mess. Perhaps you need to clean things up a bit, clarify your situation. It looks as if everyone is willing to help.'

This is an example of the working group where the members are really trying to understand and help the protagonist understand the nature of his dilemma. The director, here, uses the trust that John has in the strength of his relationship with the director, to encourage the group to be open and challenging in a spontaneous way. Following Yalom's (1975) principle, the director counts on John's experience of genuine concern for him to allow this forceful interpretation to be speculated upon in this dramatic way. Looking closely at his response it is obvious that the protagonist has 'heard' some of the messages contained within the doubling, but not all by any means. It was some time before John accepted the nature of his collusive relationship with his mother and reacted to its implications. But as director at the time I was delighted at the boldness and perception of the group members, evident in the doubling. I decided that perhaps the next time we worked with John we would look at his relationship with his father.

The group as a container

The group acts as a container, boundaried by time, place and membership. The containing promotes safety and trust. In such a place risks can be taken, strong feelings of love and hate can be expressed, and indeed, catharsis may occur. Sometimes these feelings are towards interpersonal relations in the outside world, sometimes towards relationships in the group and sometimes towards the intrapsychic feelings that arise within individuals. Here, of course, I am assuming continuity and persistence in the life of the group. I am well aware that some groups are transient and unstable in terms of membership. If that is so then it represents a restriction of the therapeutic possibilities of the group.

Containment is a very important therapeutic idea. It is no more than commonsense to realize and accept that, as human beings, we need to find safe repositories for painful ideas, feelings and experiences. Sometimes, paradoxically, those who are closest to us in our personal lives are so embroiled in these experiences that they cannot safely contain on our behalf; on the contrary their own needs may well invalidate such a position. Fortunately a well-conducted psychodrama group allows its membership to share intimate feelings and ideas without the intense embroilment of family life, with its sexual aspects and tensions of hierarchy and caring.

In analytic groups (Foulkes, 1975) there is an assumption, based upon the problems of intimacy that I have described, that members of the group will desist from any form of ingroup sexual relations. So a strong, safe and supportive therapy group, working in a spirit of 'abstinence', may well be the most appropriate setting for psychological work, which has, potentially, an undermining or destructive character attached to it.

In individual therapy there may well be occurrences of gross emotional and physical behaviour brought to therapy and tested against the acceptance of the therapist. An example of this was a clever, talented and successful young business man, married to an attractive wife, the father of a young boy child, working with me in individual psychotherapy, who regularly had recourse to prostitutes. He was especially attracted to a particular group of prostituting women, who related to each other in a complex manner, sometimes supportively, sometimes competitively. This situation was held as a secret from his wife, family and friends although a few colleagues at work had been speculating about his sexual life. It was obvious that he needed a secure, confidential arena in which to explore the meaning of his activities as well as a relationship that would contain his deep feelings of anger, guilt and anxiety. In this instance it was the trust in the relationship with me, his psychoanalytic therapist, that encouraged him to work with integrity, but it might have been trust in a group setting. Certainly, acceptance with a group of peers would have been very reassuring to him. He regarded himself, frequently, as almost beyond contempt. Interestingly enough one or two of the prostitutes showed more understanding for his plight than he did. They frequently tried to reassure him concerning his essential worth as a human being. In this context it is worth remembering Yalom's (1975) curative factors that I addressed earlier in this book and how appropriate they would have been to this young man's needs.

A range of roles

A further task of the group is to give members an opportunity to play a range of roles, some of which are very unfamiliar to them. They are, in this way, educated in the ways of the world. For example, in the case referred to above, some rather judgemental members would have gradually come to understand and find common appreciation of the place of prostitution in our sexual world and how important it is, whether in the case of heterosexual or homosexual desire. By playing the part of prostitute and speaking from that role, with assistance from the protagonist and more experienced members, the individual concerned would be informed in a manner that they had never anticipated. Their prejudices and lack of experience would have previously stood between them and the need to understand, before judgement is made.

My own view is that the learning value of psychotherapy is often underestimated, or at least not given sufficient attention when evaluating the process. As a director I have frequently been presented with social and psychological material that has been beyond my own immediate experience. In this instance the group has been a setting in which to learn. The director is informed, too, by the interplay of psychological forces in the group, which influence the roles played. Partly the evidence is in the choice made by protagonists, when casting their life dramas, and the response of members to that choice. More evidence comes in the form of doubling. Who doubles and with what insight and influence is often of great interest to the director.

The director is not the only person witnessing and processing these choices and their outcome, in terms of activity within the psychodrama. Gradually the group membership will build up a repertoire of experience of each other as the weeks go by. It is from this experience that new dramas will emerge and new material will be explored the members gaining confidence in one another as new depths of exploration are plummeted. Zerka Moreno responded, when asked to describe and evaluate the therapeutic values of psychodrama, by stating quite straight forwardly that psychodrama is 'a non-punitive laboratory for learning how to live' (quoted in Kellermann, 1992). I like this emphasis upon learning, which supports the view of the psychodrama group as being a learning environment.

It is interesting that Kellermann (1992) himself writes challengingly about the way that psychodrama and its process and aims have been viewed over the years from Moreno to the present time. Moreno, he points out, has described psychodrama within a number of frameworks of reference. Sometimes as a theology (Moreno 1920), sometimes as dramatic art (1923), sometimes as a political or social system (1953), a research method (1953) and a method of therapy and a practical philosophy of life. Obviously any psychodrama director/practitioner can attach herself to any of these concepts and find ways of implementing their position throught the practice of psychodrama. Kellermann settles for a more modest definition: 'a specific method of psychotherapy, a treatment approach to psychological problems'. My experience is that most clients I have worked with, in the National Health Service or in private practice, look to psychodrama in the terms described by Kellermann. The group they have joined has largely supported that way of looking at psychodrama and has incorporated it into their group culture. In this respect the growth of the group analytic movement has been most influential in a creative and supportive way.

The group's own business

By this I mean that the members have an active part to play in examining and reflecting upon their existence as a group. Blatner (1973) has some interesting observations to make about this activity. It accords with my own view, which is that the group should be afforded the dignity and maturity to be encouraged to confront and comment, sometimes through action, on the social, professional and clinical life of the group and how it is affected by the behaviour of individual members or subgroups. There is no doubt that subgrouping can and will, in certain circumstances, take place. Blatner suggests the *spectogram* as a way of examining such phenomena. This is easily done by using sculpting and symbolic posture and positioning to describe feelings that arise in a group when subgrouping or individual splitting takes place. Imagine a member who, angry and disillusioned, decided to leave the group. The group is distressed about this decision and is encouraged to strike up a sculpt to illustrate their varying feelings of anger and loss at the thought of the member leaving. The director simply asks the group to leave their chairs and stand up within the circle, the chairs having been pushed back, but still in place, outlining the parameter of the group. The member who is leaving the group positions herself in the circle in relation to the group as a *whole*. Then the rest of the group are asked to place themselves in a position that reflects their own feelings about her departure. Distance and closeness are used here as a measure of emotional involvement. The director can go further. She can prompt the members to *strike a pose and gesture* that shows dramatically this emotional feeling. This achieved, the leaving member is invited to respond. She may do this simply in a pose or she may speak to the group in the here and now of the action. Sometimes this feedback comes in the sharing moments of the closure. In a similar situation I once introduced the idea of the 'door', the 'way out' as it were, as the reference point for all concerned. It neatly dramatized the notion of leaving and going away, possibly never to return.

In this chapter we have been discussing the way that people *work* in the psychodrama group, whether it be a clinical or a training group. By work what is meant is identifying with the aims of the group, learning to co-operate with colleagues or patients in the group, acquiring the skills required to be a good contributing group member, and understanding that the group is not there to simply gratify individual needs but to respond to the demands of individuals through careful consideration, evaluation and exposure, through which psychotherapeutic learning can take place. This lifts the function of the group member to participant therapist in the life of the group alongside the skilled and trained therapists who will also be present. This challenges the psychiatric model of mental health, but supports the view of Moreno in his vision of the group members as active agents of investigation and change.

Chapter 11

The unities of time, place and person

The unities are expressed in therapeutic arrangements such as boundaries, confidentiality, membership, loyalty, trust and the pursuit of ethical principles. These issues of principle and purpose are examined in this chapter.

Every student of the humanities will recognize the classic principles of the artistic unities as expressed in the title of this chapter, but it is not the intention for the chapter to explore aesthetics and their relationship with psychotherapy, although it is arguable that there is a relationship, in the broadly humanistic view of the nature of psychotherapy, as an aspect of our culture and as a life enhancing activity. Rather I am concerned to stress the significance of the unities when they are seen as part of the proper arrangements for effective group psychotherapy.

Time

Time is, in part, an invention of men and women, which seems to be an essential ingredient of the social and psychological organization of our lives in Western Europe. Time, as well as being a universal preoccupation, plays a different part in the lives of human beings, emphasized and formed by the cultural expectations of the peoples concerned. Here in the West we seem preoccupied with controlling a good deal of our work and social experience by the strict observation of time. In psychotherapy it is generally true that most therapies place an enormous emphasis upon strictly allocated and observed boundaries of time.

Beginnings and endings

Psychoanalysis, in particular, places an almost religious emphasis upon the therapeutic hour, which turns out not to be an hour at all, but fifty minutes. The origins of this regime sometimes seem to be lost. As far as I understand it was devised as a practical management system by Freud to allow himself a 10-minute breather between patients, of whom he probably recruited a number in order to make a living as a doctor in Vienna. Freud had constant money problems.

The culture of Freudian psychoanalysis stresses time as a frame within which a special experience can be organized and a special relationship between therapist and client can be enacted. The timeframe is tightly boundaried so that the participants know exactly when it begins and ends and what belongs in the session and what does not. The same arrangement was adopted by the group analysts as they developed and became increasingly guided by psychoanalytic principles. Some schools of therapy regard this insistence on a tight inviolable structure as oppressive.

On the other hand I remember being quite shocked, in my psychodrama training experience, by the easy attitude of the therapist/directors towards the issue of time in our personal psychodrama performances. There was no declared limit to the time the psychodrama would perform. The directors were even happy to put a performance on 'hold' while we broke for a cup of coffee. On one occasion we broke off for a complete meal. This I found 'amazing', accustomed as I was to both individual and group personal therapy that was time bounded in a very strict way. I half expected something dreadful to occur – quite what I do not know, because nothing catastrophic did appear to occur and we found that we were able to get back into our psychodrama roles and performances with little difficulty. The nearest experience I had to this in the past was when I was an actor at Unity Theatre in London, where we would break from rehearsals for a coffee or lunch, and then go back into our roles. Of course, during performances that went on for weeks at a time we would hold our roles from one performance to the next without difficulty. The comparison is flawed of course. As actors we were only carrying within us roles that had been created in the imagination from a given script. In psychodrama we carry within us roles that are created by the living experience of actual human beings. Nevertheless I found it helpful to recall the experience when I first encountered this apparent flexible approach to time, an approach that challenged all my previous therapeutic training experience. It will challenge some readers of this book I imagine.

It should be remembered that here 'training experience' is being described. The training group was invariably experienced as completely self contained. Typically the group would meet for a weekend, in a residential setting, where the only business of the group was to work in psychodrama. The group was essentially in a bubble of time that excluded everything, except the experience of psychodrama and the needs of training. In our everyday experience, of course, this is not the case and living in a Western culture we are bound to time schedules that require us to conform. There is work to be done, salaries and wages to be earned, families to be reared, and relationships to be maintained.

For the most part clinical work in psychodrama is going to take place in the context of other demands upon our time and attention, whether we work privately, in our own setting, or in an institutional one. In a letter to a clinical director of a National Health Service therapeutic community who had asked for some guidance on the setting up of a psychodrama service in his community, I suggested to him that a whole afternoon would be appropriate, on a weekly basis, giving the therapists and patients about three to four hours to work with. Some of that time would be needed for a therapist–co-therapist debriefing, at the end of the session, assuming formal supervision would take place on another occasion. This seemed to me the workable minimum to employ in planning the therapeutic encounters in a week of work in such a community.

What is implied here is the significance of regular and continuous work in psychodrama for the patients in this community. I am not assuming that all the patients would be in this therapy group or in parallel psychodrama groups but it is probable that the assumption would be that the patients would be offered a block of time to use the membership of the psychodrama group to best advantage. This is where the psychodrama group is part of an integrated approach to therapy within an intensive community structure.

Of course a psychodrama group may well be offered as outpatient therapy. This sometimes means a once-a-week meeting in a continuous, permanent group with a slow changing membership. It is likely that the group will meet as an evening session with time limiting the duration of the group in a controlling way. In practical terms if the group starts at about 7 p.m. then it will probably close at about 10 p.m. So here the directors need to establish a ritual that will easily fit into this frame. At first it will seem very restrictive but experience shows that a good working group will get quickly down to work and easily carry the culture and the history of the group from week to week. In this respect it is like the analytic group, where good therapeutic habits are quickly established and a culture develops that becomes good habit.

How long should a psychodrama group exist? How long is a piece of string? In the example given above the psychodrama group, as an outpatient provision, is a permanent group with a fluctuating membership as patients come and go. The advantages are obvious. 'Old' members inculcate 'new' members with the culture and rules of the group. The disadvantage is that a hierarchy exists in respect of experience and length of stay in the group and some 'splitting' or 'pairing' might well have to be dealt with as 'old' members cluster together to defend themselves from 'new' arrivals. 'Old' members might well be distressed to see an 'old' and valued member who has left 'replaced' with a new 'upstart' member, challenging the norms of the group. The director, too, might come under attack for promoting new membership. But all this is grist to the mill for an experienced psychodrama director with a background of analytic understanding. And psychodrama provides an excellent medium through which to work in dealing with these group tensions.

Assuming that the arrangement of the slow, permanent open group is not possible then there are other possibilities. The best, I believe, is to form a group with a lifespan of about one-year, meeting, as far as is practically possible, once a week for about three hours a week. In this case a closed membership is probably the best arrangement, where the whole membership of the group can go through the formative and developmental stages of the group together, becoming a good working group. The completion and disbanding of the group would then be experienced by the whole membership in common.

Other formulations are possible and sometimes less frequent but more intensive periods of work are attempted; for example, the weekend workshop or daylong group. The possibilities are pretty well endless and for training groups are often quite appropriate, but I remain convinced that the steady work of the weekly group, with a known membership, is the best formulation for creative clinical and training work. It might be said that *time is then the essence of the contract.*

Place

The group may meet anywhere. In the letter to the therapeutic community director I spoke about the 'place' meaning the physical presence of the psychodrama studio in his proposed building. I was concerned with dimensions, availability, control, atmosphere, equipment, decoration and furniture. I was proposing the ideal in the knowledge that there would, inevitably, be compromises. The main issues are those concerned with therapy. The place has to be a safe place, both physically and emotionally. It has to be safeguarded from intrusion. I once worked for a terrible ten months in an old National Health Service mental hospital where porters and nurses thought nothing of walking into the middle of a therapy session in order to carry out some domestic or maintenance task, without any notice or 'by your leave'. After months of futile struggle to find a suitable place in the hospital to work, I ended up in the waiting room of the electroconvulsive unit with my group, who saw the funny side of this arrangement. I resigned – there was no *place* for psychotherapy in that hospital. The institution won, hands down. Our group was never safe. It was regarded with suspicion and dislike by the great majority of the psychiatrists on the staff, and the nursing staff were quite disdainful. Now this was some 12 years ago and I know that, thankfully, the situation today has changed and group psychotherapies of various kinds are practised in the National Health Service – even psychodrama is cautiously welcomed. So, in another sense of the word, there is a *place* for psychodrama in the formal treatment of mental health patients in the National Health Service.

The dramatic space where psychodrama is performed needs some description and discussion (Blatner, 1973), especially when the director is working in an institutional environment where she may have very limited control over the therapeutic milieu. Blatner describes the classical Moreno theatre, which is usually beyond the practitioner's reach. Here I will attempt a more modest, realizable, suggestion.

The ideal is a purpose-provided room. It should be between 6 m² to 8 m² with only one entrance – preferably from a corridor. The windows should be well provided with curtains and perhaps at a height that does not invite the voyeur. A window with a view is a nice idea, but not one that looks immediately upon a busy thoroughfare. A first-floor location is probably the best for privacy, with access to light and a view through a window. The room should be well endowed with wall sockets and some interesting lighting, including a few spotlights – definitely *not* strip lights, unless they are against a wall and firmly shielded. Some basic sound equipment is a must, together with microphones and simple sound recording gear. Today a TV and VCR together with a decent video camera, mixer and robust stand are certainly desirable features. Furniture needs to be light and simple: easily moved seats and some low tables together with rugs and large cushions are desirable objects to support the dramas to be performed. I suggest a props box with all sorts of bits and pieces of clothing, sheets, towels, old telephones, typewriters and so on, that can be used imaginatively in performance. A rakish hat can turn a rather respectable, dullish man, very quickly into a possible rogue! The possibility of varying working levels is excellent if it can be achieved. Special rostra can be bought to achieve this, which I prefer, rather than a fixed raised stage. A friendly stage designer from the local repertory theatre might offer advice and information.

It is important to give the studio a sense of being a warm, friendly working environment, and a few attractive plants, flowers in season, decorative pottery and interesting pictures on the walls go a long way to giving the psychodrama space character. Unfortunately most of our institutional provision, in hospitals and day centres, where a psychodrama group may well be on offer, are often poorly designed or adapted and aesthetically unattractive, equipped with poor quality furniture and unimaginative furnishings. The psychodrama studio can be an island of physical interest in such a setting where the staff use their spontaneity and imagination to provide a truly therapeutic space – a place of hope, adventure and change. Within this safe space I suggest that the psychodrama may ritualize its performance to the benefit of the individuals in the group and the group as a whole. Imagine the group gathering. They pull their chairs into a fairly close circle. The psychodrama director has hers and as she sits she notes who wishes to be near her in the circle, perhaps flanking her on either side. The group begins to talk in a friendly manner, gradually getting more serious and approaching the issue of who is going to be chosen to be the protagonist. A decision is taken. At this point it might be that the director chooses to swap chairs with a group member to sit beside the intended protagonist to commence an interview from a sitting position. The group is still in a relatively small circle. Then, perhaps at the director's suggestion, the protagonist gets up to continue the interview within the circle but in a new position. A position of movement. The group quite automatically begins to open up. Chairs are pushed back to create the acting space but the circle of safety and action is still preserved. The advantage to the members of the group is that they are anticipating their own performance as auxiliary egos. From this position they can enter and leave action easily. This is psychodrama in the round, not in the proscenium arch.

The director in an institutional setting might find herself having to defend her territory against intruders and takeover bids. In one hospital I know, an attractive studio, purpose built for drama therapy, was taken over by a manager for business meetings, or used for individual one-to-one therapy by a clinical manager. The creative therapists were helpless to resist this. It needed firm action from a senior member of staff to save this territory from misuse, and this action was not forthcoming. The psychodrama studio, by its very presence, incorporates a simple repeatable ritual that holds the group together in a common purpose, with common values and ways of being.

A private working studio, along the lines I have described, exclusively within the management of the psychodrama director, obviously provides a desirable milieu to work in. Unfortunately very few therapists have the financial means to provide such a setting privately. I suppose Virginia Woolf's cry for: 'a room of one's own and a thousand a year' still resonates to this day. A word of warning. Established freelance directors, who are often recognized trainers, are sometimes asked to run a residential training weekend in psychodrama. Apart from the intrinsic interest in the work there is often an attractive financial inducement. The director/trainer can find herself saying yes, unconditionally and quickly, without much information to go on. Then comes the nasty surprise when arriving at the venue to find it unworkable.

Some years ago I offered an experiential workshop, using psychodramatic methods, to a large, important conference of professional psychotherapists. I specified to the organizers the space and facilities I required, which I deliberately kept to a workable minimum. On arrival at the conference centre, a Cambridge college, I went to inspect the room allocated to me. It was about 12' long and 8' wide and full of chairs! I had offered to work with a group of about 14 members. About 16 turned up and we sat cheek by jowl to each other as I attempted to work with spontaneity and therapeutic imagination in this oppressive setting. So freelance directors – be warned and, like the Boy Scout, be prepared.

Person

People make up the membership of the psychodrama group. Who are they? Does selection have any place in the process of membership? Should a therapy group be balanced in the Foulkesian (1975) sense? Barnes, Ernst and Hyde (1999) discuss this at some length. They point out the advantages of the balanced group where there is not just *one* young woman, or *one* black person, or *one* gay man, or *one* unmarried middle-aged single man or woman. While this seems good sense and desirable, it remains very difficult to achieve where referrals are uncertain and there is no pool of waiting patients or clients, who want to come to group therapy, present in sufficient numbers to achieve this kind of balance. The writers also discuss the contra-indications for group work and feel that it may be possible to select *in advance* of admission to the group people who will 'find the group unbearable and those whom the group find unbearable'; the same criteria are attached to issues of trust. They discuss the potentially disruptive patient and the threatened individual. Clearly all these categories are likely to produce severe difficulties for the therapist/director of a psychodrama group, but the problem is that the selection methods available to us are notoriously uncertain and fraught with subjective perceptions on the part of the selectors (Feasey, 1999). Some of the characteristics described as being undesirable may not come to be known to the director of the psychodrama group, or its members, until the group is formed and launched into being as a working group. I was quite amused at the idea of the person who, they state, might be the one the group finds 'unbearable' – the truth is this person is only likely to emerge in the group as a result of the group composition and relationships. So the 'unbearableness' has to be addressed in the context of the group. Trying to discover it in advance is probably not likely to be a fruitful exercise.

A pre-group admission interview is probably desirable for the formation of a clinical psychodrama group. Clients deserve to be informed as well as assessed and the interview should be as much concerned with this function as with clinical suitability, which remains a doubtful area (Feasey, 1998). The psychodrama director will be able to offer pre-group activities that help new members to get the feel of what membership of the group might be like. Even an individual, coming for a one-to-one interview, can be drawn into a simple warm-up exercise by the interviewing director. This provides more information, experientially, than dozens of descriptive words.

A new group, coming together for the first time, can be invited to take part in simple group dramatic activities that offer a flavour of what it might be like to be in the psychodrama group. A pleasant, but challenging activity, to help new members get a feel for dramatic work, is to offer them a chance to work with the 'magic shop' technique.

The possibilities for development are endless and the technique not only provides a good exercise in fantasy and the use of metaphor as a means of exploring the human psyche, it also gives insight to the director and members into their life goals and the possible outcome of their choices. The members can be observed 'playing' creatively with these ideas and experiences and the shopkeeper, played with astuteness and imagination, can be the instrument for opening up new channels of thought and judgement for the members of the group. In my own experience the use of paradox is most useful in this fantasy game, where the shopkeeper frustrates and stimulates the shopper to press a case or engage in a lively barter conversation that opens up the clichés of desire to critical examination.

This creative introduction to the proposed psychodrama group seems to me to be full of possibilities for mutual assessment by therapist and client. There is a place for a more structured session where information is exchanged and the boundaries and timetabling and expectations of group membership can be discussed.

Foulkes (1975) notes in his book how psychotherapy group members quickly embrace the notion of trust and confidentiality as part of the therapeutic process of the group. I think this is true, too, for psychodrama groups. It is usually assumed, as Foulkes comments, that members will share some of their group experience with the most significant person they are in relationship with at the time – a wife, sexual partner or other close relative or intimate. But the understanding is that this will be done discretely without obvious and open revelation of the identity of the persons concerned. Most members, too, accept that they should avoid 'falling in love' with each other and pursuing an 'ingroup' sexual relationship. Inevitably people will become friendly, but they need to act with discretion and most important, bring the relationship to the attention of the group from time to time. Similarly rivalries and dislikes will occur and need to be treated in the same way. Sometimes it is the business of the therapist to draw attention to these powerful relationships and what they might mean in the context of the group. Sometimes other members of the group shoulder the responsibility.

Although we all look for comfort in our lives, it is best if the members do not eat, drink or smoke during sessions unless it is part of the drama. All of these activities in a psychotherapy group tend to be displacements, representations of otherwise unspoken needs. The best way of dealing with these needs is to bring them openly to the attention of the group through the process of the group. They should never be ignored. Unlike an analytic group which follows the principle of 'suspended action', Foulkes' (1975) psychodrama encourages action within a controlled, therapeutic analytic format, where the action is observed and interpreted by the entire group as well as the director. This makes it even more important to restrict or challenge activity that undermines therapy, as it occurs in or outside the group. Foulkes (1975) experimented with the use of psychodramatic methods in the Second World War, as a treatment method, stating that he used the material produced 'for further analysis and consideration'. However, when considering deeper issues concerning the use of action in therapy, he remained a questioning presence, admitting that other analysts were happy to employ the technique when they thought appropriate, but clearly holding on to a reserved position for himself.

People in the group have to recognize quickly that the psychodrama group is not a recreational group in the usual everyday sense of the word, although it may be enjoyed. It *is* a working therapy group where the success of the group, as a therapeutic agent, will depend upon the way the group and the individuals within it, agree to work together for their mutual benefit. Obviously, the director plays a key role in this process, but finally it is the responsibility of each and every member of the group to work within the process if creative and good outcomes are to be expected. Unlike the amateur drama group there is no ambiguity about this at all. Although the members may 'enjoy' their membership, they have to face the fact that from time to time they are individually and collectively going to experience discomfort and pain.

This is where and how the *person* and *persons* come together in a *time* and *place* for a purpose – the purpose of psychotherapy through the medium of psychodrama.

CHAPTER 12

The psychoanalytic presence

'Essentially, one might say, the cure is effected by love.'

Letter from Sigmund Freud to Jung, 6 December 1906.

Throughout the book I have been referring to the conscious mind and taking its presence for granted in the mind of the reader and what might be described as the general public. We wake in the morning and until we sink into slumber at night, we are connected with the world around us and all our relationships through the perceptual apparatus of the conscious mind. When we go to sleep we enter another realm, the function of which remains in dispute but the character of which is beyond dispute. We enter the realm of the unconscious, the world of dreams.

Moreno never disputed the presence of both these states of being. This is not really an issue. What is more difficult to establish is the relation of one to the other and how each might influence the content and mental process of each. In psychodrama it is perfectly possible to pursue the work of therapy without taking much cognizance of these dilemmas. Indeed, many good trainers and practitioners would probably look askance at my concern. But this book is attempting to offer analytic perspective to the work of the psychodrama psychotherapist and with that aim in mind it is necessary to allow some time to discuss what might prove to be interesting issues.

The dream state of sleep provides absolute evidence of the unconscious mind and it should be of interest to psychodramatists that much of our dreaming, but not all, takes the form of dramatic narrative. It is not necessarily very coherent or well put together but, nevertheless, invested with feeling. Conflict, anger, pleasure, fulfilment, frustration, confusion, and erotic experiences are only some of the more common states of feeling we enter into, accompanied by a suitable *dramatis personae* to play out the appropriate story where one is present.

The argument among psychologists is: what is the purpose of this nightly activity? Our observable rapid eye movement (REM), as we sleep, tells the observer that dreaming is taking place. But what is to be made of the content and structure of the dreams? The psychologists remain in dispute about the nature of dreaming. The most reductionist view is that it is no more than the brain simply ridding itself of what might be described as unwanted material in the mind. Rubbish! I mean that in both senses. It is thought of as 'rubbish' but I think that conclusion is 'rubbish'!

When Freud wrote *The Interpretation of Dreams* (1975b), he described dreams as offering us the 'royal road to the unconscious'. He felt then that this was perhaps the most important book he had written up to that time. I agree with him. In psychoanalysis the dream is valued. Perhaps more in the past than now. It is difficult to quantify the use of dream material in psychoanalytical work. In psychodrama, although I have worked with dream material offered by clients, I realize that it was unusual. Athough I have read about, witnessed, performed in and directed many psychodramas, it occurs to me that I have not seen much attention given to dreams. The literature is sparse on the topic. I will return to this particular concern at a later point.

What are thought, memory and visualization, together with imagined action, doing in the unconscious mind? Is the unconscious mind as separate from the conscious mind as is sometimes supposed? We know that the ideas appear to float into the conscious state that do not have immediate environmental stimulus. We catch ourselves thinking about someone, or a past happening, or a future expectation in circumstances that do not seem at first sight to be connected with the conscious state that we were in, until these thoughts and imaginings occurred. In a recent Melvyn Bragg interview on television, a young film director remembered how surprised he was when he reproduced, in a film set, an interior of a teenage boy's bed room – a room that almost exactly mirrored his own when a boy! All done without conscious intention. A psychoanalytical psychotherapist would certainly not be surprised at what had taken place. The deeply invested memory of childhood and adolescence had asserted itself in a context that made sense, the dramatization of the world of an adolescent character, within a drama, where the room held great significance as a place of retreat, comfort, exploration and fantasy. In a sense it could be argued that the film director had 'acted out', but here it is quite obvious that it had a benign character about it; in fact the memory was used creatively, without any conflict, in the designing of the set for the film. This supports my contention that the unconscious is not merely a repository for anxious ideas and experiences – it can and does hold a storehouse of valued memories and deepest desires.

The psychoanalytic presence 137

Freud (1975c) wrote of what he described as the 'psychopathology of everyday life'. He treats all the small examples we experience of the unintended and 'accidental' as being of significance, often as examples of the unconscious mind active in our interactions with the world about us. My view is that this is not so much an intellectual mental process but rather an emotional intervention within a given context of thought or action.

The following is a small example of something occurring like this in a psychodrama when the protagonist, a young woman, was going to her mother's flat for an important emotional encounter.

Scene 39

A psychodrama training group, well established and of some standing.

Director: 'So Mary, you are going to your mother's flat. How do you intend to get there? Or perhaps you want to open the scene in the flat with her?'

Mary: 'No, I think it would be nice to walk there. I don't want to hurry it. I want time to think. Her flat is about 10 minutes walk away, down the hill and around the corner.'

Director: 'OK. Shall we start?'

Mary: 'Fine.'

They start to walk around the stage area together quietly reflecting upon the coming encounter with mother. After a while the director asks her if they have walked enough, whether she feels OK to approach the flat.

Mary: 'Yes, I'm OK it's just around the corner, here.'

At this point Mary suddenly stops and looks surprised. She virtually freezes.

Director: 'What's happening Mary? . . . she pauses . . . What's in your mind?'

Mary: 'Oh my God, my sister Jean is there. I can see her at the bottom of the street. She is standing outside the flat.'

The director takes a quick decision and beckons to an auxiliary woman player/therapist to take up a position just ahead of Mary. Not looking at her, apparently not noticing her, staring at an imaginary door.

An unexpected figure has entered the scene. But she is a figure of great emotional importance and her presence is apposite. No, Mary is not suffering a psychosis. Her visualization of her sister at this moment is a contribution from her unconscious mind. The director makes the figure concrete through the medium of the auxiliary, in order that Mary can now make a decision as to whether to keep the character in the psychotherapeutic frame or not. She can choose whether to use the experience or not. In this particular instance Mary recovered her poise, found some emotional energy and freedom, and with some force responded.

Mary: 'Oh push off, Jean, it's just typical of you to try to get into the act and it's typical of me to let you. But not this time. I am going to talk to mother alone. We, you and I, Jean, can talk later and we will.'

As the protagonist, Mary in this instance, is familiar with and valuing the presence of the unconscious mind in her life, she allowed the moment of visualization, when she called up the image of her sister, so spontaneously and without any fear, to enter briefly into the psychodrama. This makes sense, for all performers and directors know we are operating in the world of 'as if' when a psychodrama is performed, where the drama shares that quality with dreaming and fantasy. Most importantly the director supported her by calling an auxiliary into action.

From this it can be deduced that the conscious mind and the unconscious mind are more subtly in connection with each other than might be supposed. A dialogue might be seen as taking place, where emotionally appropriate responses are possible. Freud, thinking and writing in hierarchical terms, stratified the mind into conscious and unconscious. He thought, too, of the unconscious mind as being somehow 'below' consciousness, a repository of the unacceptable thoughts and feelings of the man or woman concerned. This applied, so he thought, especially to sexual introspections, fantasies, memories and reflections. Repression was seen as a mental mechanism of defence. But contemporary thinking would see the unconscious mind as playing a more dynamic part in conscious life, with positive elements of influence where the recipient of influence responds with interest and insight to the presence of such interventions even when they are, as in the instance of the psychodrama described, unexpected and spontaneous.

I have likened the psychodrama performance to dreaming. At this point it is worth looking briefly at the approach to dreaming that may be made within the context of the psychodrama. Kellermann (1992) discusses what he calls an 'intrapsychic' procedure, which he suggests 'explores the internal world of the self'. In this procedure the protagonist identifies 'parts' of herself or 'important aspects' of herself that can be almost discretely identified and seem to enter into intrapsychic flows of communication. Then, using the empty chair technique, these facets are localized and addressed both separately and together. This links with many views about the nature of the dream. The view is that the dream state is essentially showing us aspects of the 'ego' in conflict or alliance, attack or defence. Thus the dream is an intrapsychic representation. However, what interests me is that, in the contemporary literature concerning psychodrama, little seems to be said about the significance of dreams or any special regard given to special techniques that may be associated with the exploration of dreams through psychodrama.

Drawing on my own experience I have described an approach that takes up the point that dream material is often associated with aspects of the ego. Thus a room, a colour, a scene, a person or persons, an animal, a piece of furniture may easily be making a statement in the dream state about the manner in which the conscious and unconscious mind explores the ego. In the instance I have given I have described the empty chair technique, which necessarily fragments the aspects. Another approach is simply to work at the narrative level of the dream whilst at the same time recognizing its symbolic and metaphorical importance.

Scene 40

A well-established training group. Dagmar, a psychotherapist, is working with dream material. Her dream was very simple. She was walking down a long, leafy, green pathway, full of natural life, overflowing with colourful leaves mostly in shades of green, towards a bower where there was a decorative seat in the classical style – it, too, surrounded by a delightful environment of verdant growth.

In this instance the director discusses how Dagmar might work with the material. She decides, with the director's support, to simply recreate and enter the dream scene again in her drama. As she does she begins to freely associate to the images and ideas that come into her mind as she enters the scene. She is delighted with the pathway, which she sees as fertile and fecund. It is leading her towards the bower.

Dagmar: *'It feels quite exciting on this path. It is leading me towards the bower. Something awaits me there, I know. I feel fruitful and as if I am part of nature, not the way I usually feel, dashing around all the time in the Fiat – I hardly have time to breath. But this feels good and I am not at all afraid.'*

Director: 'Can you associate the path with any part of your body or being?'

At this point another member of the group, a big man, begins to fidget in the group. He wants to double. But the director holds him back with a gesture. Dagmar doesn't appear to notice this activity on the edge of her space.

Dagmar: 'Well, it is a bit like I imagine it must be like inside me sometimes. You know I am a woman and I could . . . [she pauses] . . . well not on my own of course, I could.'

She stops.

The man in the group is getting more fidgety.

Director: 'You could. You could, what?'

Dagmar: 'Oh I don't know. It's really very silly. I couldn't possibly have a baby now it would be ridiculous. I need a good partner.'

The man in the group is now more relaxed and has stopped fidgeting on his chair.

Director: 'And the bower?'

Dagmar: 'Oh it's lovely.' [She giggles.] 'Well, I suppose it could be my womb! I will get there eventually, I am sure I will.'

Director: 'It looks as if that is where you want to go, doesn't it? And you would obviously hope the journey is going to be a good one.'

Eventually Dagmar reached the 'womb'-like bower where she encountered her present boyfriend and began to work with him on the issue of commitment and her desire for a child.

Naturally the interpretation of this dream could have been immensely varied. Here the director is following the cues provided by the protagonist. He asks her to *freely associate*, a technique identified by Freud in his earliest days of work and discovery, as a method for reaching the unconscious mind.

Notice, too, some overspill into the group. The man in the group suddenly had a feeling he wanted Dagmar to be pregnant. A strong nudge from his unconscious stirred him into wanting her to represent his own desire for fertility. He needed to be contained and restrained from expressing his own libidinous drive in that particular context, although, at another level, the director was well aware of his intuitive response to her fallopian imagery. In this context the dream is shared by the group so such resonance should not be regarded as unusual.

I have given two approaches to working with a dream, but these approaches are in no sense exclusive, and a great deal depends upon the imaginative energy of protagonist and director alike, in finding a way of working that best suits both.

Freud wrote revealingly about the manner in which the unconscious penetrates to our conscious world through mistakes or misunderstandings. We trip over ourselves in such situations and sometimes we ruefully acknowledge this happening. Sometimes it simply makes us angry and frustrated. At best it amuses us. The most obvious examples are slips of speech, which may immediately create embarrassment for us and others. In a recent biography a former assistant to a Labour MP at the House of Commons found himself, to his discomfort, calling the MP 'dad'. A client of mine recently confessed to telling her son, not once but twice, on public occasions when meals were being eaten, that he was getting fat. She said: 'I just found myself blurting it out. He was terribly upset, I even said it about him to a waitress in a restaurant.'

Sometimes we become blind. In one analytic group in which I was a patient the analyst looked around for a moment and asked 'Helen, any one know where she is?' She was, in fact, sitting in the group in her usual chair at the time. The group responded with silence and Helen began to weep, quietly and angrily. As a group therapist I have sometimes been checking the numbers sitting in the room, members of an outpatient psychotherapy group, and found I couldn't get the numbers to add up to the same each time I counted! In another group, where I was a patient, a member of the group would regularly fall asleep, snoring gently. The group would ignore it as if it wasn't happening. The group analyst waited patiently for our response, which was, effectively, to be deaf and blind in denial. My feeling now was that he might well have helped us in a simple interpretation of our situation given to us as a reflection on our 'blindness' – our eyes were apparently shut too, perhaps 'not seeing the wood for the trees'.

I have noticed in psychodrama that group participants seem a little unwilling to confront such mistakes as if they do not wish to produce shame and anxiety in the perpetrator, especially if it is the protagonist. I suppose it is a form of inhibition brought about by projective identification.

Body language, too, plays its part. How often a client in an individual session, striving to be open and frank, suddenly closes her arms across her body very firmly as if to say 'thus far I go but no further'. In psychodrama it is common for the protagonist to suddenly become almost physically frozen, inept and clumsy. The protagonist cannot think what to do next, or how to respond, and the body behaviour reflects with great accuracy, the internal position of conflict and ambiguity of purpose. I was almost ashamed on one occasion when my co-therapist in a psychodrama intervened, literally pulled me briefly away from the protagonist, an attractive young woman, and hissed into my ear in his laid back Californian accent and manner, 'give her room man, give her room'. I had no sense of my close proximity to her at the time, absolutely none. We must have been only inches apart. In that moment, which had protracted into more and more minutes, my body behaviour was revealing that of which I was quite unaware, in any conscious sense. All these instances of involuntary behaviour, often shown in body language, need to be observed, briefly acknowledged within the director's perception, and sometimes, if rarely, drawn into the action.

The same applies to mistakes made by the protagonist in setting up a scene. I can think of some rooms I have seen created without a door either to get into the room or leave. Sometimes all that is called for is the director to draw attention to the absence of such an obvious feature missing and unaccounted for. Furniture sometimes appears in such quantity that there is no room to move or is absent in telling ways. Often the paradoxes are quite amusing, as if the unconscious mind is having a little joke, illustrating the depth of the contradictions, normally not acknowledged. There is of course a wonderful play called *The Chairs*, by Ionesco, a piece of theatre of the absurd based on this phenomenon, which exploits this idea in a frightening and black comic manner.

This chapter is necessarily only offering a very partial view of the influence that psychoanalytic ideas may have upon contemporary approaches to psychodrama. Freud, here, is attributed with much of the definitive influence, but the early pioneers of psychoanalysis who worked alongside Freud and eventually parted company with him, have their own contributions to make. An early psychiatrist and psychologist and enthusiastic supporter of Freud in the foundation period of psychoanalysis in Vienna, was Alfred Adler. Freud's discoveries and formulations concerning the nature of the unconscious proved very attractive to him although he was, and remained, sceptical throughout his life concerning the centrality of sexual anxiety as a prime cause of neurosis. Through a mixture of ideological tension and personal rivalry he parted company with Freud in 1911 and set up a school of thought of his own, which focused upon the social impact of interpersonal relationships as definitive formulating experience in the life of human beings. Freud was very angry with him for his desertion of the 'cause'. Adler especially identified the notion of the 'inferiority complex' and its accompanying compensatory complex that offers a rather vulgar and ineffective show of confidence, not so much spoken of in our own time. The term has been somewhat abandoned now – we talk of a 'loss of self esteem' and 'painful feelings of inadequacy'. This language is very familiar to the psychodramatist of our time. Again we notice that people experiencing these disabling feelings often make unsuccessful attempts to dress themselves in a cloak of unconvincing confidence.

Although there is a presence of Adler in this country it is probably true to say that Adler's influence has been much more profound in America where he held a chair in psychology at the Columbia University, New York City in the 1930s. However I believe that psychodramatists in the UK would do well to take note of his views and teaching.

Another major psychoanalytic figure who broke from his association with Freud is Carl Jung. Jung remains influential in the UK although there has been much splitting and rivalry among his British followers. Jung is a controversial figure for a number of reasons. His split from Freud again focused upon the issue of sexual anxiety. However, there was much more to the fissure. Jung himself had always been attracted to the mystical and religious and this contrasted strongly with Freud's determined atheism. Jung's special contribution has been to the understanding and nature of symbol and myth, especially as revealed in dream associations and psychotic or psychological fantasy. He formulated a concept of the *collective unconscious* made up from what he describes as *archetypes*, primitive images associated with human experience and the large issues of life and death.

As far as the psychodramatist is concerned much of this disputable material is probably of small significance; however, Jung's respect for the 'spiritual' aspect of the human experience will resonate with many protagonists within the drama who will sometimes require support in their struggle to understand themselves and their relationships in aspects that go beyond the immediately psychological. Dramatherapists, in particular, frequently find that the client's personal journey works well, therapeutically and energetically, when associated with a traditional story (myth) that elaborates deep issues of life and death. They have a respect, too, for ritual, which, as a psychodramatist, I have attempted to incorporate into the life of psychodrama treatment and training groups. This may be no more than focused starting and closing with repeated meaningful statements, rituals and social gestures.

I would like to close with a brief discussion of the work of Melanie Klein, who has perhaps intruded into the English scene of analysis with more impact than any other individual in the last 50 years. Interestingly enough she is referred to in *Encarta* (the computer encyclopedia) as an

English psychoanalyst, which, of course she eventually became by naturalization. In fact she was an analysand of Ferenci from Budapest. It could be argued that she arrived in England, rather as Freud did, pursued by the horror of Nazism in Germany and its representation in prewar Hungary by the White Guard.

In the late 1930s, London, and Hampstead in particular, was hosting a gathering of central European psychoanalysts, many of them Jewish, fleeing the prospect of persecution and even death in their homelands. So in this sense I write of Klein as an intruder into the then-Freudian (for the most part) scene of psychoanalytical thinking in London, centred around Ernest Jones, Freud's biographer. Her contribution to psychoanalytic thought and theory at the time was to posit what seems to me the improbable idea that children and babies could and did organize complex unconscious fantasies around what she described as the 'depressive position' and the 'paranoid position' – all this in the first 12 months of life. I am not sure how useful this idea would be to a contemporary psychodramatists. As a well known psychoanalyst put it:

> Unfortunately, in their formulations, the Kleinians appear to have attributed profound psychological knowledge to the infant by confounding psychological behaviour and biological behaviour . . . they endow the infant with psychological intentionality and complex cognition in the first few weeks of life.

Ironically this would appear to be a clear case of another Kleinian idea: 'projective identification' whereby complex adult mental and emotional concepts are projected towards the thinking and feeling behaviour of the baby and attributed to its inner state – an idea that I would support and I would offer evidence to validate it. Klein confounded a great deal of clear thinking about early states of psychological experience for infants, by talking about 'bad' and 'good' 'objects'. My objection to this formulation is twofold. Firstly the notion of 'bad' or 'good' being attributed to this early stage of awareness in infancy, seems quite erroneous, it even hints at a moral as well as psychological judgement. It also signifies the idea of the baby being able to 'split' off one idea and feeling from another in almost a rivalrous, or evaluative way. This is a difficult suggestion to entertain. The earlier idea from Freud of 'pleasure' and 'unpleasure' seems much more useful. Furthermore the reduction of important figures of emotion in our internal landscape to mere *objects*, or even *part objects* feels reductive and unhelpful. For the most part these internal figures are very powerful. Frequently imagined in our childhood and adult life, they are fleshed out with presence in a way that the term *object* hardly attempts to suggest. The suggestion that, for example, the infant will isolate the 'breast' in the feeding experience seems unlikely. The feeding mother will inevitably communicate so much more, as any casual observer of breast or bottle feeding may notice and record. Mother's smell, her voice, her breath, her touch, her eyes, her presence as a whole figure in the landscape of pleasure and satisfaction impacts upon the baby's sense of the world about her. But it is something of a mystery as to how these sensations are organized and integrated into the developing ego. It seems improbable to associate all these sense pleasure responses to the idea of the 'breast', in the sense that the word communicates to adult carers.

Very recently I watched an infant of two-days old snuggle and nestle against its birth mother's face while its mouth opened and appeared to seach for the breast. It was an obvious instinctive gesture. Even more interesting was the fact that, when held by another loving relative, the baby began to cry as if to signal distress at having lost the smell and touch of the mother's skin. I cannot imagine that there was any thought attached to this behaviour or any imagery constructed in the mental process of this baby. All appeared to be instinctive.

However, having made this short critique, it has to be acknowledged that Klein has had immense influence in Britain and in some parts of Europe – less so in America. Through the agency of Bion (1961) her ideas have come to be an influence in group psychotherapy. Her abstractionism seems to have a particular appeal to the English School. It seems strange, too, that the abstractions are sometimes closely linked with what seems extravagant, even theatrical terminology. The language is concerned with feelings and expressions of hate, rage, attacks, destructive envy, depression, paranoia and so on.

If the reader wants to read more about 'object relations' and psychodrama from a more sympathetic writer, then I can recommend the book on the subject by Paul Holmes (1992).

As far as the contemporary psychodramatist is concerned I believe that a sympathetic recognition should be given to the Kleinian view of the force of 'projective identification'. In the role play of protagonists and auxiliary egos, 'projective identification' is often evident, and the director has to be properly alert to preserve the integrity of the protagonist's performance. It is important for the director to know what feeling or state of mind belongs *to whom* in the process of the drama. We all know too that the internalized figures of significant people, places and experiences of the past, play an active part in shaping our present. The past lives in the present, in both a benign and malignant way, and we encounter it in the psychodrama performance. On the other hand we must also be careful to examine propositions that are sometimes attributed to Klein, and that appear to undermine the story of Oedipus, with great concern. It is a story as old as woman and man and its presence on the psychodrama stage is frequently palpable. It is supported by an ancient and classical literature. If you go too far along the path with Melanie Klein, this could become a problem.

CHAPTER 13

Ethical issues

'Art thou weary, art thou languid
Art thou sore distressed?'

Art thou Weary, Art thou Languid? tr. John Mason Neale

As with psychoanalytic psychotherapists it is incumbent upon any psychodramatist, registered with the UKCP or not, to hold an ethical position as a psychotherapist. This ethical position, in my view, embraces not only the responsibility not to actively *abuse* a client, but also to *safeguard* the client in a professional setting of proper care. The care has to be an active ingredient in the relationship between client and therapist if it is to have any value and meaning. The medical imperative is *to do no harm* and that needs to be the therapeutic position that is enacted in the relationship.

Dependency

Holmes (1992) wrote:

> I have been asked, often, by therapists with a psychoanalytic background, how it is that I can run a 'one off' psychodrama workshop and then not return to the group. They feel that I should continue to care for the protagonist. I respond by saying that such behaviour would encourage the group members' dependency on me. Eventually each of us must take (as far as possible) responsibility for our own actions and future . . . But in the end real emotional growth comes only from an acceptance of our adult independence of each other . . .
> This is an aspect of the existential philosophy of psychodrama, a philosophy that for me is in no way at odds with a psychoanalytic understanding of the human personality.

When I read this I immediately remembered John Donne's famous expression from 'Devotions Upon Emergent Occasions' (1623) 'No man is an island entire of itself . . . And therefore never send to know for whom the bell tolls; it tolls for thee.' The communitarian is very strong in me. It should be remembered, too, that Sartre's hero at the end of his existential novel, *The Road to Freedom*, chooses to commit himself to those around him in actions, which will probably cost him his life.

Paul Holmes may be satisfied with this statement but I imagine that the psychotherapists who raised the question in the first place are not, and neither am I. Interestingly enough it is the last statement in his book and I wonder if he was trying to have the last word in a difficult and contentious discussion among psychodramatists. Notice how he qualifies his statement. He uses the word 'eventually' at the beginning of the third sentence. Well how long is 'eventually'? He writes 'But in the end . . .' but when does the 'end' come? Could it be after a three-hour psychodrama with a stranger group where the members will not meet together again in that manner. Hardly likely. I think the concern of the psychoanalysts is well placed. It would be my concern too and, unlike Paul Holmes, I will not conduct such therapy in such a setting and have mounted a modest campaign to inhibit such work by psychodramatists. I hold this position partly out of my personal emotional and moral response towards my clients and partly out of my training and the culture of psychoanalysis. I am surprised that with his own background, in sophisticated psychotherapy training in the psychoanalytic field, that Paul Holmes is able to mount what appears to be a flimsy defence of the practice of 'one off' psychodrama session, followed by what could be seen as abandonment.

The worst example of this I have come across was at a British Psychodrama Association conference where a psychodramatist author, whose writing I admired, ran a workshop that I attended. A woman protagonist emerged and a short but intense piece of work was enacted. To my surprise and dismay he suddenly dismissed the protagonist from the room, without any supporting auxiliary figure, and continued to run the workshop at a discussion level. About three quarters of an hour later we all left the room and I suddenly came across the 'protagonist' sitting alone, quite obviously distressed. I was ashamed at my own failure to act in the workshop, to challenge what I believe to be unethical behaviour, or my failure to approach the woman and offer some support. I raise the issue of ethics here because I cannot support the idea that ethics only belongs in the place of gross misbehaviour, such as sexually abusing the client. Obviously the British Psychodrama Association has a professional conduct committee to which a person thus abused could take a complaint. It is a professional and responsible body. But unfortunately it is a fact that 'victims' of such professional abuse often feel guilty and responsible for their own suffering and do not recognize the need to complain. It is obvious, too, that even an experienced therapist, witnessing such behaviour, can fail to go the professional conduct committee – witness my own failure. I was intimidated by the 'stature' of the lecturer and his place at the conference. I dreaded the personal consequences if I made a fuss, interrupting and upsetting this distinguished presenter's workshop. My fear was that other persons at the workshop would turn on me in anger for 'spoiling' the workshop and attacking the presenter. It was a cowardly omission.

My belief is that ethical behaviour is woven into the best practice of the professional therapist, who is seeking the best outcome for the client and certainly avoiding, in an active sense, what could easily become damaging behaviour.

To conclude, the discussion of dependency is well known to virtually all practitioners of psychotherapy, from whatever school. Most of them respond with therapeutic approaches that deal creatively with the experience, not abandonment. There is a concept known as *working through* where the client is enabled to experience and understand the different stages of an emotional relationship in the structure of a psychotherapeutic relationship. This would clearly include the experience of dependency and attachment with all its implications for the healthy growth of human relationships. Ironically, as far as the Holmes statement is concerned, psychodrama provides an excellent context for this work to proceed on a continuing basis, where the group has some substance and continuity of being.

Kellermann (1992), discussing the frequency and duration of psychodrama sessions, takes an ambiguous position. Whilst at first justifying the 'one off' session as being productive and containing positive results, apparently from his own research material, he goes on to quote Kipper (1983) who states:

> ... such one session case reports may unintentionally convey the message that 'it takes one psychodrama session to do the job.' It is important to be cognisant of that possibility and make certain that readers will not falsely understand it this way.

A strong word of caution and reserve. Of course the group or individual analyst would never allow such an idea to enter an evaluation of an early session.

I have never come across any research material, objective, or otherwise, originating in the UK, that suggests that effective psychodrama therapy is possible in 'one off' sessions. In a therapeutic community, in which I worked, 'one off' sessions in psychodrama were experienced by community members but only within the context of ongoing small-group and large-group therapies, including dramatherapy, art therapy and relaxation therapy. Members were in the community for months at a time. In such a setting the notion of a 'one off' session is pretty well meaningless because the client is well established in a continuing group milieu.

Gratification

There is a well-known enjoinder to psychoanalytic psychotherapists to work within the 'spirit of abstinence'. This is easier said than done because all of us, whatever our occupation, look for satisfaction and gratification in our work. The more serious matter is where the psychodramatist is guilty of running a psychodrama group primarily to satisfy the self. There may be a mixture of motives present. Directors have the need for money, for professional experience, gaining qualifying hours of training experience to satisfy a training programme, to gain esteem, for praise and distinction. They may also have a drive towards the exhilaration of wielding power and influence, to feed the ego with sexual satisfaction, albeit at third hand, through the admiration and attachment of client members of the opposite or same sex. We are all human and most of us are honest enough to admit to motives that are not exactly pure. But most of us know that it is incumbent upon us to have enough self awareness to protect the client from our sometimes unhealthy appetites. Unfortunately this is not always so.

The special difficulty for the psychodramatist is that the very act and production of the drama has a performance character attached to it. Many talented directors have a performance background to their lives. Indeed I can confess to this myself. For the most part this background can be assimilated harmlessly and creatively into the talents that the director has to offer clients towards their work in the therapy. But I have been present when a director has come under strong pressure from an audience to set up a performance to 'entertain'. Then the *self-regarding need* of the director has responded. The needs of the client are subsumed to the need of the director to perform – the need then is not so much to provide a useful therapeutic experience for the audience, but rather to satisfy an inner compulsion to 'shine', to be special, to be admired, and especially to admire the self, to gaze into a mirror that reflects the self in performance and admire it. The charismatic director has to struggle with these deeply seated human needs. They are particularly burdened with the expectations of those around them, especially trainees and admiring clients. They come under pressure when they attend conferences and workshops. The conference will seek a performance, a voyeuristic experience. Therapists, especially those working in the creative arts, are especially vulnerable to this demand. Unfortunately, there are usually 'client' figures present, at such conferences, who will respond to invitations to work in front of the assembled conference. They are exposed when they actually need protection.

Persecution

The book *Lord of the Flies* by William Golding describes, in vivid terms, the primitive behaviour of a group of boys when they identify a sacrificial figure in their membership and sets out to destroy it. The book ends with 'authority' in form of a naval officer's boot standing in the sand, representing the *super ego* of judgement and control and eventually the repression that makes civilization possible. Freud in *Totem and Tabu* (1950), in *Civilization and its Discontents*, and in *Group Psychology and the Analysis of the Ego* (1975), discusses this phenomenon with great insight and persuasiveness and alerts us to the potentially destructive possibilities of the human group. It is incumbent upon the psychodrama director, even without reference to Freud, to address this issue and to be aware of the dynamics that can unleash primitive destructive behaviour in the group. The protagonist, offered as victim to the group, is an unhealthy figure. There are individuals who, from a need for punishment, will manoeuvre themselves into that position. So the dynamics are of collusive punitive behaviour, where unwitting sadistic impulses may be gratified. It should be remembered that this aggressive behaviour may express itself outwards to imagined enemies, outside the group, or inwards to enemies identified inside the group. If readers have any doubts about his human activity I would simply draw their attention to the metapsychological scene, where irrational fears and hatreds have lead to the decimation and destruction of entire tribes and peoples in last years of this century, in violence in Europe and Africa, the Yugoslav Federation war, Hutu/Tutu conflict, the war in Chechnya and slaughter in Philippines. On a smaller scale, the abuse of political/immigrant refugees in Britain, as I write this book, is being associated with a rise in racial attacks on the streets of our cities.

Emotional and sexual abuse

I can do no better than to refer readers to the excellent book by Newnes, Holmes and Dunn (1999). Pages 45 to 50 contain a worrying list of publications that are all concerned with the emotional, physical and sexual abuse of patients and clients of the mental health services in this country, some of whom, even more worryingly, have experienced these abuses at the hands of therapists. There is a growing literature in this field, especially coming from America, on the subject of seduction and sexual exploitation of women clients, usually by male therapists. I have noticed, in the culture of psychoanalytical psychotherapy in this country, there is no special emphasis upon this obvious misbehaviour. Indeed I have noticed, quite shockingly in one instance, a tendency to 'cover up' such offences when they occur and a colleague is involved. In the instance concerned there was a highly placed male therapist, steadily corrupting and seducing junior female psychotherapy staff, whilst at the same time playing the role of supervisor of their therapeutic work and training as therapists. Other senior staff knew about it, and lower levels gossiped about it, but nothing was done to inhibit his pathology until a relative of a female patient made a formal complaint of sexual abuse by this so-called psychotherapist. Not surprisingly when this 'therapist' was removed the service he controlled virtually collapsed.

For the psychodramatist this situation is unlikely to occur in such a closed and inclusive manner. Rather, if it occurs at all, it will be in the form of the 'groupie' who follows the therapist from one group to another, and who, having 'fallen in love' with the therapist, seeks emotional and sexual gratification and is encouraged in the response of the therapist. Of course, the therapist may simply fall in love with a group member. This undoubtedly happens. The only possible ethical response to this situation is, if the loved one is agreeable, for the group member to leave the group and cease to be a 'client'. If the loved one is not responsive to the therapist then the situation needs to be resolved in a different manner. It is difficult to propose the particular resolution in the absence of a real situation but it is likely that the psychodramatist would be able to restrain her passion in favour of the professional position. Supervision is the key to managing such a situation. She may need to withdraw as the group's therapist.

Tim Bond (1991), discussing the issue of sex between counsellors and clients, notices how, in the apparently simple, succinct statement of the British Association of Counselling (BAC) on ethical matters in 1984: 'Engaging in sexual activity with a client whilst also engaging in a therapeutic relationship in unethical.' There lay a number of ambiguities. Firstly was the BAC saying it's OK as long as you cease to be the client's counsellor immediately? Was the statement insufficiently rigorous? Some counsellors thought that a post-counselling sexual relationship was always inappropriate; some thought that time had to pass before such a relationship could be validated – some years perhaps. Fritz Perls (1969) was quoted in the discussion as a 'reputable' therapist, of some standing who certainly did not rule out sexual relations between client and therapist as always unhelpful and unethical. I notice that nearly 10 years later the BAC position on sexual ethics is barely changed and the injunction to pay attention to the post-counselling relationship is made in terms of supervision discussion, rather than underlined with prohibition.

The British Psychodrama Association has its own professional committee, which deals with complaints against psychodramatists. It also publishes a code of practice that is as rigorous as any other therapeutic body. But the test of such codes is in their implementation, and the instances I have quoted show it is sometimes very difficult to bring a 'rogue' therapist to book.

Emotional exploitation is always a part of sexual abuse but emotional exploitation comes in many different guises and the overtly, physical sexual element may be disguised or represented in a displaced manner. Often it takes the form, in the psychodrama group, of the most favoured client, but it might also represent itself as quite the opposite, the most unfavoured and marginalized client. These intense feelings may come from the director in quite obvious or more subtle aspects of the therapeutic relationship, but it is possible for these feelings to arise in any member of the group and they can be directed towards another member. The feelings may be acted upon in quite unconscious ways, which need to be opened up, identified, and dealt with by the psychodrama director in her role as group leader/facilitator. In addition it is for the psychodramatist to be especially alert to the presence of emotional overattachment, from herself towards, or from, any of her clients. She also needs to admit to herself feelings of rejection that may be present in her towards a group member. Hopefully these feelings will be addressed in supervision.

Emotional abuse may take place under the guise of therapeutic work where the director uses her power to persecute a protagonist under the cloak of addressing defences. The same behaviour may come from group members who, without conscious awareness of what they are doing, may 'double' in a persecuting or derisory way. Sometimes it is very difficult to decide the real intention of sarcastic or angry doubling. The correct way to deal with it is to be completely conscientious as a director in checking out the situation with the protagonist and addressing the issue in the group as the opportunity occurs.

Supervision

Just as the concept and practice of supervision is central to psychoanalytical psychotherapy and counselling, it is obvious that the practice of psychodrama calls for the professional practice of supervision to provide protection and good therapeutic experience for client and psychodramatist alike. In this respect supervision becomes more than a technical issue and moves into the area of ethical practice. The issues discussed in this chapter would all be properly addressed in the supervision process.

CHAPTER 14

What next?

In this short chapter I set out how to go forward to training as a psychodramatist, how to gain experience as a potential trainee, and how to get psychodrama as psychotherapy, to meet your own personal needs. They are all intertwined.

To deal with the first question first

There is no compulsory registration of psychotherapists in Britain, including psychodramatists, and it is possible to learn to become a competent psychodramatist from a number of 'unauthorized' sources. I trained with the International Foundation for Human Relations in Miami. However, it is probably best to follow a relatively safe and regulated route to training, qualification and registration through the auspices of the British Psychodrama Association and its associated training bodies. Listed below are the addresses of the organizations concerned, from which you can make a start. You will have to choose your training organization. They are all regarded as competent by the BPA and I imagine, for most people, it will be as much a matter of geography as anything else when it comes to a final choice. Individuals may wish to shop around and meet the trainers face to face before making a final choice and investing money as well as time in what will probably prove to be a lengthy process.

Hoewell International
Psychodrama Centre
North Walk
Lynton
North Devon
EX35 6HJ
(contact Marcia Karp and Ken Sprague on 01598 753754)

London Centre for
Psychodrama and Group Analytic
Psychotherapy
15 Audley Rd
Richmond
Surrey
TW10 6EY
(contact Jinnie Jefferies and Olivia

Lousada on 020 8948 5595 – note that this body is not formally associated wth the Group Analytic Society)

Newtown House Centre
Doneraile
County Cork
Ireland
(contact: Catherine Murray on 00 353 22 24117)

Northern School of Psychodrama
Glebe Cottage
Church Rd
Mellor
Stockport
SK6 5LX
(The Registrar 01436 831200)

The Jesmond Centre for Psychodrama and Counselling
9, Stratford Grove,
Heaton'
Newcastle on Tyne
NE6 5AT
Director: Jenny Biancordi
(telephone 0191 265 9664)

This centre, whilst not providing a full qualifying diploma, is useful for its provision of introductory training and experience.

Oxford Psychodrama Group
8 Rahere Rd
Cowley
Oxford
OX4 3QG.
(contact Peter Haworth and Susie Tylor at 01865 715 055).

South Devon College
Department of Music and Theatre Arts
Newton Rd
Torquay
TQ2 5BY
(contact Dorothy Langley at 01803 217 551)

For more information about the British Psychodrama Association contact:

James Scanlan
The Administrator
Heather Cottage
The Clachan
Roseneath
Helensburgh
G84 0RF
(telephone 01436 831 838, email www.zambula.demon.co.uk)

This organization has recently published an informative booklet.

For a more cosmopolitan training experience conducted mostly in continental Europe contact:

Doreen Elefthery
Director
The International Foundation for Human Relations
10891 SW 67th Avenue
Miami
Florida
33156
USA

For readers who just wish to obtain some experience in psychodrama in a practical way, it might be a good idea to join the BPA as an interested person. Through that membership they will certainly be drawn into the network of short courses and weekend or day-long offerings in psychodrama that are on offer from various sources. It is likely, too, that trainers associated with the training bodies I have indicated will offer these introductory experiences.

For readers looking towards psychodrama as the personal therapy of their choice, it is more difficult. I think the best place to start is with your nearest registered trainers who will probably know where such a group, private or NHS, may be found. The UKCP Register is the preferred guide. Alternatively, if there is a psychotherapy centre near at hand, again either private or NHS, then an enquiry through them might produce results. If such a group is available then it will probably be run in the early evening, on a once weekly basis, associated with an outpatient provision. If offered in the NHS then it will be free on referral from a doctor/psychiatrist. If it is a private group then fees will be charged. These are very variable but can be as much as £20 per person per session. A *careful* advance enquiry is recommended.

There is a growing library of psychodrama texts available in this country and the bibliography in this book points to the best. All of them are available, by request, from your local library.

And finally, don't forget the Internet. Just type in the word 'psychodrama' on a search site and wait!

Closure

The actors, holding hands, step forward to take their bow.
The director emerges, modestly from the wings.
The curtain closes . . . slowly.

Bibliography

Barnes B, Ernst S, Hyde K (1999) An Introduction to Group Work. London: Macmillan.
Bion WR (1961) Experience in Groups. London: Tavistock.
Blatner A (1973) Acting In. New York: Springer.
Blatner A (1988) Foundations of Psychodrama. New York: Springer.
Bond Tim (1991) Ethics for counsellors. Changes: An International Journal of Psychology and Psychotherapy 9(4): 204–93.
Brazier D (1994) A Guide to Psychodrama. Constable: London.
Brecht B (1998) Messingkauf Dialogues. London: Routledge.
Brown JAC (1950) Social Psychology of Industry. London: Penguin.
Burton J. (1955) Drama in School. London: Jenkins.
Casson J (1997) British Journal of Psychodrama and Sociodrama 1/2: 7–18.
Culpan FM (1979) Studying action sociometry. Group Psychotherapy, Psychodrama and Sociodrama 1(32): 122–7.
Davies B (1975) Use of Groups in Social Work Practice. London: Routledge.
Davies MH (1988) In Group Therapies in Britain. Milton Keynes: Open University Press.
Dryden W, Davies B, Feasey D (eds) (1972) Working with Youth. London: BBC Publications.
Feasey D (1998) Will it or won't it work. Changes: An International Journal of Psychology and Pscyhotherapy 16(2): 92–104.
Feasey D (1999) Good Practice in Psychotherapy and Counselling. London: Whurr.
Foulkes SH (1948) Introduction to Group Psychotherapy. London: Heinemann.
Foulkes SH (1957) Group Psychotherapy. London: Pelican.
Foulkes SH (1975) Group analytic Psychotherapy. London: Interface.
Freud S (1950) Totem and Taboo. London: Routledge.
Freud S (1975a) Group Psychology and the Analysis of the Ego. London: Pelican.
Freud S (1975b) The Interpretation of Dreams. London: Pelican.
Freud S (1975c) Psychopathology of Everyday Life. London: Pelican.
Gale D (1995) What is Psychodrama? Loughton, Essex: Gale Publications.
Holmes P (1992) The Inner World Outside. London: Routledge.
Holmes P, Karp M (1991) Psychodrama Inspiration and Technique. London: Routledge.
Ionesco E (1956) The Chairs. London: Nelson.
Janov D (1970) The Primal Scream. NewYork: Putnam.
Jennings S (1973) Models of practice in dramatherapy. Dramatherapy 7(1): 3–6.
Kane R (1992) Research in psychodrama. American Journal of Psychotherapy, Psychodrama 44(2): 168–172.

Kellermann PF (1992) Focus on Psychodrama. London: Jessica Kingsley.
Kipper DA (1983) Book review. Group Psychotherapy, Psychodrama and Sociometry vol. 36: 193–201
Martineau RF (1989) JL Moreno. A Biography. London: Routledge.
Matthews J (1966) Working with Youth Groups. London: ULP.
Merei F (1994) Group leadership and institutionalisation. Human Relations 2(1): 23–9.
Molnos A (1987) British Journal of Psychotherapy. Quoted in Psychodrama Instructions and Technique. Homes Karl: Routledge
Moreno JL (1923) The Theatre of Spontaneity. New York: Beacon.
Moreno JL (1934) Who Shall Survive. New York: Beacon.
Moreno JL (1941) The Words of the Father. New York: Beacon.
Moreno JL (1946) Psychodrama and Group Psychotherapy. New York: Beacon.
Moreno JL (1957) The First Book on Group Psychotherapy. New York: Beacon.
Moreno JL (1959) Paper in Journal of American Society for Group Psychotherapy and Psychodrama Vol 12.
Moreno JL (1972) In Journal of Group Psychotherapy, Psychodrama and Sociodrama. New York.
Moreno Z (1964) The First Psychodramatic Family. New York: Beacon.
Newnes C, Holmes G, Dunn C (1999) This is Madness. Ross-on-Wye: PCCS Books.
Nicoll A (1955) World Drama. London: Harrap.
Perls F (1969) In and Out of the Garbage Pail. Lafayette, Calafornia: Real People Press.
Quin BJ.(1991). In Holmes P and Karp M (eds) Psychodrama Inspiration and Technique. London: Tavistock.
Rogers C (1969) Two Divergent Trends. New York: Random House.
Ryle A (1976) Group Psychotherapy. The British Journal of Hospital Medicine. March 1972.
Sacks JM (1995) Bibliography of Psychodrama. New York: Beacon.
Satre J-P (1945) The Road to Freedom. Penguin Modern Classic. London: Trilogy.
Schutz W (1975) Encounter. In Corsini R (ed.) Current Psychotherapies. Itasca, Illinois: Peacock Pubs.
Schutzenberger A (1975) Psychodrama, creativity and group processes. In Jennings S (ed.) Creative Therapy. London: Pitman, pp. 131–56.
Skynner R (1974) Group Therapy. In Varma V (ed.) Psychotherapy Today. London: 233–249.
Slavson SR (1943) Introduction to Group Therapy. New York: Harvard University Press.
Widlake B (1997) Barbara's bubbles. The psychodrama of a young adult recovering from an eating disorder. British Journal of Psychodrama and Sociodrama, vols 1 and 2: 23–41.
Wilkins P (1997) Psychodrama research. British Journal of Psychodrama/Sociodrama 1/2: 44–60.
Wilkins P (1999) Psychodrama. Sage: London.
Williams A (1989) The Passionate Technique. London: Routledge.
Willis ST (1991) In Psychodrama Inspiration and Technique. London: Routledge.
Winnicott D (1971) Playing and Reality. London: Tavistock.
Yalom ID (1975) Theory and Practice of Group Psychotherapy. New York: Basic Books.

Index

abuse, emotional and sexual, 151–153
action
    as benefit of psychodrama, 48–50
    levels, 56
    moving into, 56, 70–73
    suspended, 48–49
Adler, Alfred, 142–143
admission interviews, 132
American Society for Group Psychotherapy and Psychodrama, ix, 7
analyst, director as, 83–84
anxiety
    about director's attention, 27
    about psychodrama, 40–41
    resistance and, 72
applications of psychodrama, xiv
artist, director as, 79–80
audience, 18
auxiliary/empty chair, 91, 139
auxiliary egos, 55
    closure, 74–75, 88–89
    groups work 119
    warm up, 69

Barnes, B., 131
benefits of psychodrama, 46–51
Bion, W.R.
    Klein and, 145
    pairing theory, 62
    therapist–client relationship, 117
Blatner, A.
    doubling, 94, 98

    group's own business, 123–124
    integration of psychotherapies and psychodrama, 22, 23, 24
    place for psychodrama, 129
    professional relationship, 58
    research, 45
body language, 141–142
Bond, Tim, 152
boundary keeper, director's role, 88
Brazier, David, 30
Brecht, Bertolt, 3, 32, 93
British Association of Counselling (BAC), 152
British Psychodrama Association (BPA), 30
    contact details, 156
    ethical guidelines, 44, 79, 152–153
    experience, 157
    professional conduct committee, 148, 152
    training, 29, 155
British School of Psychoanalysis, 104
Brown, J.A.C., 35
Burton, Jim, 3

case history, 46
Casson, John, 44
catharsis, 16–18, 57
    learning, 37
    Moreno on, 32
Charcot, Jean-Martin, 16
Clarkson, Petruska, 28
closed groups, 16

closure in sharing, 56, 74–75
  process of director, 88–89
cognitive learning, 29, 41
  directors, 33, 35
collective unconscious, 143
confidentiality, 57, 133
conscious states, preoccupation with, 51–52
container, group as, 121–122
continuing professional development, 45
corrective emotional experiences, 106
countertransference, 16
  group psychotherapy, 23, 27–28
Courtney, Tom, 3
Coward, Noel, 2–3
Culpan, F.M., 21
cult of the personality, 78

Davies, Bernard, 6, 117
defensiveness, 41, 52
delusional states, 54
dependency, 147–150
dependency in group, 27
depression, 54
depressive position, 144
de-roling, 74–75, 91
descriptive nature of psychodrama, 48
diagnostic tool, psychodrama as, 46
diagrammatic description of psychodrama, 55
  director, 57
  ethics, 57
  five instruments, 55–56
  notes, 56–57
  professional relationship, 58–59
  technique, 57
director, 55, 57, 77–78
  as artist, 79–80
  closure, 74–75
  countertransference, 28
  doubling, 97–98
  group needs, primacy of, 51
  group psychotherapy, 21, 24–25
  group work, 117–118
  as interpreter and analyst, 83–84
  interview, psychodramatic, 98–99
  as leader, 78

learning, 29, 30–36, 77
  group work, 118
  sources, 155–157
  support, 111–113
  as the memory, 82–83
  moral, 78–79
  process of, 86–89
  professional relationship, 58–59
  protagonist, emergence of, 65–66, 67
  as psychologist, 84–86
  relationship with client, see countertransference; tele; therapist–client relationship; transference
  resistance, 72, 106
  safe, 81
  sculpting, 100
  as strong woman, 80–81
  support for protagonist, 111
  talking in the group, 61, 62–63
  transference, 26–27, 58–59
disempowerment of group, 27
displacement activities, 133
doubling, 94–98
  group work, 119
  unconscious material, role of, 52
drama, 2–4
dramatherapy, 2, 143
  games, 63
dreams, 135–136, 138, 139–140
Dreikurs, Rudolf, 58
Dunn, C., 151

ego, 139
'ego' psychology, ix
Elefthery, Dean, 7
  group psychotherapy, 14, 52
  on needs, viii
Elefthery, Doreen, 7, 156
emotional abuse, 151–153
emotional learning, 29
  directors, 35
empty/auxiliary chair, 91, 139
enabling distance, 89
encounter, vii
encounter groups, ix
ending groups, 127–128
equipment needed for psychodrama, 53, 129

Index

Ernst, S., 131
ethics, 57, 79, 147
    dependency, 147–150
    emotional and sexual abuse, 151–153
    gratification, 150
    guidelines, 44, 79, 152–153
    persecution, 151
    supervision, 153
exhibitionist therapies, ix
existential model of psychotherapy, 59
experience, gaining, 157
expression of feelings, 48

families, 50–51, 56
favouritism of directors, 27
fear of director's attention, 27
feedback stage, 56
feelings, expression of, 48
Ferenci, Sandor, 104
Foulkes, S.H., 2, 5
    groups, 131, 133
    origins of psychodrama, 57, 103–104, 133
    on psychodrama, 11
    suspended action, 48–49
    therapist–client relationship, 116, 117
    transference, 8
free association, 140
    and spontaneity, links between, xv, 57
Freud, Sigmund, viii
    acting out, 115
    arrival in England, 144
    catharsis, 16–17
    countertransference, 28
    cult of the personality, 78
    dreams, 136
    family life, significance of, 56
    on Ferenci's views, 104
    followers, need for open-mindedness, x
    free association, 140
    influence, ix, xiii
    Jung and, 143
    Moreno and, 6–7, 9, 103
    mothering and fathering, 102
    persecution, 151
    pleasure and unpleasure, 144
    psychologist, director as, 86
    resistance, 41
    time, 126
    transference, 13, 21, 24, 58
    unconscious, 52, 137, 138, 141, 142
frozen action, 97

Gale, Derek, 30
Golding, William, 151
gratification, 150
group, 55
    as container, 121–122
    group's own business, 123–124
    lifespan, 127–128
    primacy of needs, 51
    as protagonist, 66
    psychotherapy, viii, 11–28
        development of group, 35
        encounter, vii
        Moreno, 5, 6, 9
        unconscious life of groups, 6, 7
    roles, range of, 122–123
    talking in the, 61–63
    work, 115, 116–118
group analytic movement, 12, 118

historical overview, 1–9
Hoewell International, ix, 155
Holmes, G., 151
Holmes, Paul, 30, 145
    dependency, 147, 148, 149
Hudson High School for Girls, USA, 6
humanistic school, ix, 117
Hungary, 104
Hyde, K., 131
hysterical paralysis, 17–18

identification, projective, 144, 145
immediacy of psychodrama, 46–48
improvisation, 63
individual psychodrama, 5–6, 43–44, 115–116
inferiority complex, 142–143
inhibition, 141
integration of psychodrama and other psychotherapies, 21–22, 23
International Foundation for Human Relations, 155, 156
Internet, 157

interpreter, director as, 83–84
interrelationships within group, 62
interventions, 118
interviews
  admission, 132
  psychodramatic, 98–99
intrapsychic procedure, 138–139
Ionesco, Eugene, 142

Janov, D., 103
Jennings, Sue
  curative factors, 16, 18–19
  group process and dynamics, 12
  improvisation, 63
  learning, 28
Jesmond Centre for Psychodrama and Counselling, 156
Jones, Ernest, 7, 144
Jung, Carl, viii, 143

Kane, Roberta, 44
Karp, Marcia, ix, 30, 88
Kellermann, P.F., 30
  countertransference, 16
  dependency, 149
  intrapsychic procedure, 138
  psychologist, director as, 84, 85, 86
  role playing, 103
  support of protagonists, 111
  transference, 13, 14, 24–25
  views of psychodrama, 123
Kempler, Walter, 58
King, Gillie Ruscombe, 89
Kipper, D.A., 149
Klein, Melanie, 104, 143–146

leader, director as, 78
learning, 28, 37–42
  by directors, 29, 30–36, 77
    group work, 118
    sources, 155–157
    support, 111–113
  role playing, 103
  value of psychotherapy, 122–123
lifespan of group, 127–128
limitations of psychodrama, 43–46, 51–54

London Centre for Psychodrama and Group Analytic Psychotherapy, 155–156

magic shop technique, 63, 132
Martineau, R.F., 9, 21–22
Matthews, Joan, 6
memory, director as the, 82–83
Merei, F., 104
Miller, Arthur, 2
mirroring, 99
Molnos, A., 104
moral director, 78–79
Moreno, J.L.
  anxiety, 72
  audience, 18
  catharsis, 16
  charismatic personality, 78
  complexity of performance, 32, 35
  conflicts, 7, 9
  encounter, vii
  followers, need for open-mindedness, x
  Foulkes' knowledge of, 2
  Freud and, 6–7, 9, 103
  groups, 6, 9, 119, 124
  individual psychotherapy, 44
  influences on psychodrama, xiii, 9
  interpersonal therapy, psychodrama as, 19
  Kellermann on, 123
  large audience psychodramas, 67
  moral director, 78–79
  origins of psychodrama, viii, ix, 57
  place for psychodrama, 129
  process of director, 88
  protagonist, group as, 66
  psychoanalysis undermined by, 85–86
  psychotherapeutic debate, 21, 22
  role playing, 4, 5, 103
  role reversal, 91, 92
  social atom, 63–64
  social construct, humans as creatures of, 83
  sociometrics, 21
  spontaneity, 119
  tele, 13, 25, 33, 58, 111, 116
  unconscious, 135
  writings by and on, x–xi

Index

Moreno, Zerka, 7, 78, 123
Mosak, Harold, 58

Newnes, C., 151
Newtown House Centre, 156
Northern School of Psychodrama, 156

object relations theory, 104, 144–145
'one off' sessions, 147, 148, 149–150
open groups, 16
Oxford Psychodrama Group, 156

pairing theory, 62
paranoid position, 144
people, 131–134
Perls, Fritz, 152
persecution, 151
personality, cult of the, 78
person-centred psychotherapists, 87
physical contact, cultural differences, 108
place of group, 20, 53, 128–131
power struggles within group, 27
process of director, 86–89
projective identification, 144, 145
props needed for psychodrama, 53, 129
protagonist, 55, 101–113
   choice of, 119
   closure, 74
   emergence, 63–68
   group as, 66
   interview, psychodramatic, 98, 99
   process of director, 87
   relationship with director, see countertransference; tele; therapist–client relationship; transference
   resistance, 72–73
   warm up, 69
psychic stages, 56
psychoanalysis, 135–146
   emergence at same time as psychodrama, ix
   influence, xiii, 6–8
   tension between psychodrama and, ix
   terminology, xiii–xiv
psychologist, director as, 84–86

Quin, Barbara Jean, 117

rapid eye movement (REM), 136
registration of psychodramatists, 29, 36, 155
research, 44–45
resistance, 40–41, 72, 106
   process of director, 87–88
resolution, 41, 50–51
resources, 53, 129
   provision of, 119–121
rites of passage, 74
rituals, 68, 143
rivalry within groups, 27
Rogers, Carl
   followers, need for open-mindedness, x
   influence, ix
   professional relationship, 58
   tele, 33, 58
role playing, 4–5, 101–104
role reversal, vii, 91–93, 103
   warm up, 69
Ryle, Anthony, 20

safe director, 81
Sartre, Jean-Paul, 148
Schultz, William, 58
Schutzenberger, Anne, 68, 102–103
sculpting, 99–100, 109, 124
sexual abuse, 151–153
sexual relations within group, 121–122, 133
Shakespeare, William, 3, 93
Shakespeare in Love, 4
sharing, *see* closure in sharing
Sing Sing Prison, 6
size of group, 20
skills learning, 29, 41
   directors, 33, 35
Skynner, Robin, 9
Slavson, S.R., 6
sleep, 135–136
soap operas, 3
social atom, 64
social group work theory, 6
socializing process, 63
sociometry, viii, 21

sociopathic states, 54
soliloquy, 93–94
South Devon College, 156
space, *see* place of group
spectograms, 124
spontaneity, xv, 57, 119–121
Sprague, Ken, 30
stage, 55
strong woman, director as, 80–81
suitability for psychodrama, 53
supervision, 153
    countertransference, 28
    emotional and sexual abuse, 152
suspended action, 48–49

technique, 57
tele, 13–14, 25–26, 116
    action, moving into, 72
    director's role, 57
    learning, 37, 41
    professional relationship, 58, 59
    training, 33, 111
television soap operas, 3
therapeutic alliance, *see* tele
therapist–client relationship, 116–117, 121
    importance, 28
    working alliance, 72, 86
    see also countertransference; tele; transference
time, 125–128
time-consuming nature of psychodrama, 53
timing of psychodrama, 32
    group psychotherapy, 20
    limitations of psychodrama, 52
tracking, 82, 95
training, 11–12, 37–42
    British Psychodrama Association, 29
    directors, 29, 30–36, 77
        group work, 118
        sources, 155–157
        support, 111–113
    leadership, 21, 36
transference, xiv, 7–9
    action, moving into, 72
    closure, 89
    director's role, 57

group psychotherapy, 13–14, 21, 23, 24–27
    learning, 37, 41
    professional relationship, 58–59
    training, 32, 33
trust
    professional relationship, 58, 121
    within group, 133

unconscious, xiv
    collective, 143
    in groups, 6, 7
    lack of focus on, 51–52
    psychoanalysis, 85, 135–142
    role, 52, 59
United Kingdom Council for Psychotherapy (UKCP)
    continuing professional development, 45
    ethics, 79
    register, 29, 36, 157

Vanier, Jean, vii
voyeurism, 66

warm up
    activities, 63, 132
        for doubling, 98
    period, 56, 68–70
Widlake, Bernard, 40–41
Wilkins, Paul
    research, 45
    tele, 58
    transference, 58–59
Williams, Anthony, 30
    resolution, 50–51
    transference, 7–8, 9
Willis, S.T., 106
Winnicott, D., 104
working alliance, 72, 86
working through, 149

Yalom, I.D.
    curative factors, 18–19, 122
    therapist–client relationship, 116–117, 121
    transference, 7, 9, 26, 58